The WHEEL of HEALING with AYURVEDA

Companion Workbook

MICHELLE S FONDIN

Copyright © 2015 Michelle S Fondin
All rights reserved.

ISBN: 1499193343
ISBN 13: 9781499193343

CONTENTS

PREFACE   vii

AN INTRODUCTION TO HEALING   ix
   Gratitude Leads Me to Healing   xii
   Acts of Kindness Chart   xiii

CHAPTER ONE A Deeper Look at Ayurvedic Mind Body Types   1
   Vata Dosha   1
   Pitta Dosha   3
   Kapha Dosha   5
   Combining the doshas if you are a two-dosha type   6
   The Pitta-Vata Type   6
   Signs that Vata should be balanced first   6
   The Vata-Kapha Type   7
   Signs that Kapha should be balanced first   7
   The Vikruti Test   7
   Interpreting Your Vikruti Test   11
   Exercise: Your Current Symptoms   11
   Your Dosha Balancing Plan   12

CHAPTER TWO A 15-Day Exploration of Dharma   15

CHAPTER THREE Physical Health Part One: Dosha Specific Diets   23
   The Vata Pacifying Diet: Promote Calm and Serenity   24
   Key Points to Keep in Mind When Preparing a Vata Meal   25
   Create Your Own Vata Meal Plan   26

The Pitta Pacifying Diet: Remain Cool and Calm 27
Key Points to Keep in Mind When Preparing a Pitta Meal 29
Create Your Own Pitta Meal Plan 29
Kapha Pacifying Diet for Weight Loss 31
Key Points to Keep in Mind When Preparing a Kapha Meal 32
Create Your Own Kapha Meal Plan 33
Weight Loss for All the Doshas 35

CHAPTER FOUR Physical Health Part Two: Daily Routine and Exercise 37

My Ayurvedic Daily Routine 39
Daily Exercise 40
My Exercise Plan 41

CHAPTER FIVE Physical Health Part Three: Detoxification of the Body 43

Panchakarma and Ayurvedic Fasting 46

CHAPTER SIX Spiritual Health: Connecting Daily 47

Living a Spiritual Life Daily 50
My Plan to Honor My Spiritual Self 52

CHAPTER SEVEN Emotional Health & Healing Your Past 55

My Day Emotionally 56
My Stress Management Strategy Plan 56
Learning From Your Past and Most Recent Past 58
The Only Limitations are the Ones Within Your Mind. 59
Lifting the Limits 60

CHAPTER EIGHT Relationship Health 61

My Love Letter to Myself 63
My Love Letter to My Potential Self 63
A Love Letter to My Most Significant Relationship 64
Allowing Your Loved Ones to Shine Bright 65
The Magic Paper 65

Contents

CHAPTER NINE Occupational, Financial and Environmental Health   67
Using Visualization and Vision Boards to Create Your Life   68
A Picture is Worth a Thousand Words   69
Adding Your Intentions and Desires   69
My Intentions and Desires   70

CHAPTER TEN Ayurveda Q & A   71

CHAPTER ELEVEN Simple Meal Plans for Vata, Pitta, & Kapha   77
Vata Pacifying Breakfast Choices   77
Vata Pacifying Lunch Choices   78
Vata Pacifying Dinner Choices   78
Vata Pacifying Snacks   79
Pitta Pacifying Breakfast Choices   79
Pitta Pacifying Lunch Choices   79
Pitta Pacifying Dinner Choices   80
Pitta Pacifying Snacks   80
Kapha Pacifying Breakfast Choices   80
Kapha Pacifying Lunches   81
Kapha Pacifying Dinners   81

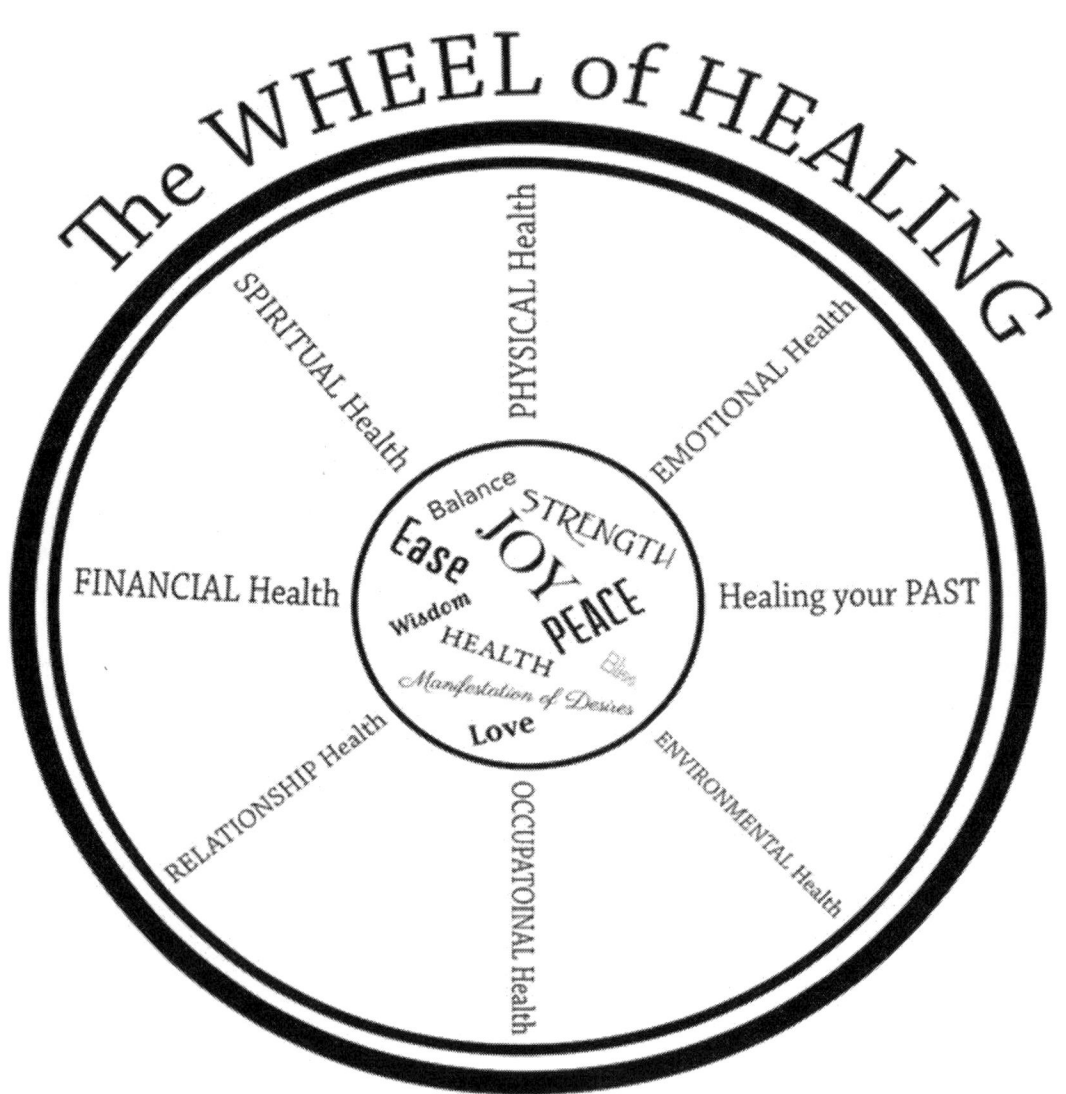

PREFACE

Welcome to The Wheel of Healing with Ayurveda Companion Workbook! You've enjoyed reading *The Wheel of Healing with Ayurveda: An Easy Guide to a Healthy Lifestyle* or maybe you bought both books at once and want to make sure your immersion into an Ayurvedic lifestyle is sound.

This *Companion Workbook* will take you in depth into each chapter of *The Wheel of Healing with Ayurveda* with additional exercises; a more expansive view of the *doshas* and more resources including dosha specific meal plans to help you include aspects of the Ayurvedic lifestyle quickly and easily.

Just like the book you can use the *Companion Workbook*, in conjunction with the *The Wheel of Healing with Ayurveda* corresponding chapter, in any order you choose. Perhaps one aspect of your life is shouting out for healing more than another right now. We have a Q & A section at the back of the book to answer questions you may be having about living an Ayurvedic lifestyle or balancing your mind body. *The Wheel of Healing with Ayurveda* approach is meant to be easy, logical and practical to your already busy life. If you find you need more structure, you can also purchase our audio set, which is designed to guide you more fully.

There is information contained in *The Wheel of Healing with Ayurveda*, which is not in the *Companion Workbook* and vice versa. So it's important that you read the book first to gain an understanding of the chapter before completing the exercises in the workbook.

Make sure you take ample time for each section and the exercises within. These are truly transformational and you'll be thankful you've set aside time to work through them thoroughly.

Wishing you a wonderful journey into Ayurveda and perfect health always.

Namasté,

Michelle S. Fondin

AN INTRODUCTION *to* HEALING

We begin with an Ayurvedic definition of health versus the Western definition. But before we explore, let's get your look on health.

1. What is your earliest memory of health or what it means to be healthy?
   _____
   _____
   _____
   _____
   _____

2. What is your earliest memory of ill health or what it means to be sick?
   _____
   _____
   _____
   _____
   _____

Now let's fast forward to today and get your concept of health now. Keep in mind that your concept is yours and there is no right or wrong answer. In order for you to feel healthy or sick, it's important to know where your parameters lie.

3. For you, what does it mean to be healthy? (Examples: *I have to be exercising four days per week to be healthy.* Or *I have to never get sick to be healthy.*)
   _____
   _____
   _____

_____
_____

4. And what does it mean to be sick or have lack of health now? (Examples: *To be sick means I have to take medications daily.* Or *To be sick means having cancer or heart disease.*)

_____
_____
_____
_____
_____

Now that you are aware of your definitions of health and illness, we will begin to shift our mindset into an Ayurvedic way of thinking about health.

Ayurveda is an all-inclusive science. It includes and embraces all healing modalities. However, Ayurveda does not take a single approach to a symptom or diagnosis as Western medicine has a tendency to do. Western medicine is extremely useful in acute cases of disease and trauma, but it's not helpful in detecting the root cause of illness from a multifaceted perspective. For example, a Western physician may determine that the cause of excessive bleeding through the rectum is colon cancer but the same doctor would have a hard time explaining why the cancer started in the colon in the first place. An Ayurvedic physician would understand that excessive bleeding is *Pitta* (*fire and water*) in excess striving to come out of the body and that *Vata* (*space and air*) normally sits in the colon. A tumor in the colon would indicate excess *Kapha* (*water and earth*). Removal of the tumor and chemotherapy might correct the cancer's growth for a time but it doesn't solve why there was excess Kapha and Pitta in the colon to begin with. An Ayurvedic physician would take a look at the person's diet and exercise regime, whether or not the person has a spiritual practice, what his emotional and relationship life is like, what type of job he has and if he's happy in his work and may even go so far as to read his birth chart.

As you can see, by this example, Ayurveda has many more tools to get to the root cause of illness. The skeptic in you may be asking, "Well, what if you can't get to the root cause?" Or "Good people get sick all the time?"

I've heard these questions before and have been humbled by the diagnosis of a close teacher of mine, Dr. David Simon, who self-diagnosed his own brain cancer and passed away only eighteen months later. You are correct to ask. We do not always have the answers. And yes, good people, who are doing the right thing, do get sick and die. There are a percentage of illnesses, in certain cases, where root cause is difficult to detect. Sometimes we have to simply trust in our higher power or divine energy because we can't see the bigger picture. Ayurvedic medicine explains we have past karma from previous incarnations that we might have to *repay,* so to speak. My teacher, Dr. Simon, was a great person, in my opinion, who lived his life according to his teachings of wellness and Ayurveda. Why he got cancer and died so quickly still baffles many of his friends and family to this day. But I trust that I don't know the bigger picture.

That being said, in most cases, over 80%, we can go to the root cause of illness. Sometimes, if the disease is well advanced, we may need medical intervention before treating the real problem. And that is what happened in my case. I first had to have two surgical procedures to remove my thyroid and encapsulated tumor and radioactive iodine therapy before doing the work necessary to get to the root cause of my thyroid cancer.

Wherever you are in your journey to health, please take a moment to get a snapshot of where you are now, today, as you read this. Please take a look at the diagram of The Wheel of Healing on page 4 and assess which areas of your life need balancing. Write them down.

Areas, which need balancing from the wheel:
_____
_____
_____
_____
_____

Now that you've written down which areas need to be balanced, prioritize them. Figure out which is number one, two, three etc.

After this chapter, decide which area you'd like to heal first. Try not to overwhelm yourself and take on too much at once. Chances are, when you begin to work on one area, others will balance out much faster.

Make a time commitment to each area; give yourself a week, a month or sixty days to balance out one spoke of the wheel. If you have a difficult time following through, give yourself a number of minutes in a day you will commit to working on your healing.

I commit to spending _____ hours/minutes per day on myself to heal.

I commit to spending _____ days on each area of healing.

Gratitude Leads Me to Healing

Having gratitude for what we have in life is a great way to start your path to healing. Often, when we focus on what's wrong or what we don't have going for us, we lose sight of what's right. Take some time now to list all of the things you are grateful for.

Your health, body, mind, emotions:
_____
_____
_____
_____
_____

Family, friends, neighbors, colleagues, teachers, leaders:
_____
_____
_____
_____
_____

Work, play, hobbies, abilities and talents:
_____
_____
_____
_____
_____

Material possessions: house, car, money, books, etc.
_____
_____
_____
_____
_____

Spirituality, connection to your universal source, peace, nature
_____
_____
_____

_____
_____

Anything else you are thankful for...
_____
_____
_____
_____

Acts of Kindness Chart

When you are feeling poorly or that your progress is not going according to your timeline, take a moment and perform an act of kindness for yourself and for someone else. It can be something simple such as offering yourself or someone else a flower. Take a moment to jot down a few acts of kindness you can do easily when you find yourself in sadness, anger or self-pity. It's even better when the person receiving has no idea of the giver. The healing for you is in the act of giving. It matters not whether you receive thanks or acknowledgement. But make sure you perform an act of kindness toward yourself first. That will leave you with more energy to give.

Acts of Kindness for Me	Acts of Kindness for Someone Else

CHAPTER ONE

A DEEPER LOOK *at* AYURVEDIC MIND BODY TYPES

In The Wheel of Healing with Ayurveda, we touched on the doshas. We will now expand our knowledge of each dosha in order to further understand our work on ourselves. I will give a textbook example of each mind body type. Since most people have mind body constitutions that are split between doshas, most will not resemble a single-dosha type, but rather see qualities of two or perhaps all three doshas.

Vata Dosha

Vata types are comprised of the elements of space (*akasha*) and air (*vayu*).

Qualities of Vata	When Balanced	Out of Balance: Mind	Out of Balance: Body
Dry	Creative	Worried/anxious	Dry skin/eyes
Rough	Excitable	Too many thoughts	Constipation
Moving	Happy	Nightmares	Insomnia
Unpredictable	Talkative	Fearful	Gas/bloating
Cold	Enterprising	Forgetful	Excessive weight loss
Light (weight)	Entertaining	Psychosis	Arthritis
Changing	Adaptable	Hallucinations	Cold hands/feet
Clear	Clairvoyant	Paranoia	Tremors

When you think of a Vata type, think of the words *movement* and *change*. Vata types are constantly on the move. They fidget, pace and get up and go all day long. They may even move in their sleep. Their energy is a nervous type of energy. They will certainly pace while talking on the phone, doodle while listening to a lecture or tap their foot if sitting at a table. Highly creative, the Vata type will have a plethora of new ideas, always. They love to try new things, buy new things and invent new ways of doing things. But rest assured, they will not hold onto something for long. They may try a new idea for a short time until another thing catches their attention, then they are off to the next idea. If you're thinking, this may make a Vata type unstable, you're right. A true Vata type changes jobs, relationships, and locations often. They may be referred to as free-spirited.

The endearing qualities of a Vata type is that they smile and laugh easily, often tell jokes, and have the playfulness and the innocence of a child.

One thing you must keep in mind, however, is that each of us has all three doshas in our mind body constitution. So while the changing nature of Vata may give you the picture of someone who is irresponsible and sometime downright flakey, know that a stereotypical Vata type is rare. You or someone you know may exhibit qualities of Vata but may also have a certain amount of Pitta or Kapha to counterbalance the airiness and spacey nature of Vata.

Pitta Dosha

Pitta types are comprised of the elements of fire (*tejas*) and water (*jala*).

Qualities of Pitta	When Balanced:	Out of Balance: Mind	Out of Balance: Body
Hot	Warm	Critical/ judgmental	Skin rashes/ acne
Light (bright)	Bright eyes	Angry/ bad temper	Acid reflux/ heartburn
Moist	Goal-oriented	Stubborn	Irritable bowels
Intense	Good leaders	Overindulgence/ addictions to food, alcohol, drugs	Skin hot to the touch/ sweating/ high temperature
Penetrating	Strong appetite	Jealousy	Body odor
Oily	Good digestion	Seek perfection	Early balding
Sharp	Sharp memory/ intellect	Workaholics	Over-sensitivity to light

The words for Pitta are *metabolism* and *transformation*. Pitta types have a medium build and very good digestion. They are the leaders in society and enjoy professions of prestige and power. The fire element gives them drive and motivation to: achieve goals, seek perfection, and go to the top of everything they do. As a result, they often burn the candle at both ends and wind up with ailments due to overwork and too much stress. Pitta types can be classified as a type "A" personality. They love knowledge and the accumulation of facts. They enjoy being right and sharing their knowledge with others. Their warm gaze attracts others as they often have beautiful eyes and a sharp look. Pitta types enjoy the finer things in life, dress nicely and strive to wear only the finest jewelry or drive an expensive car. They are often bright but can also be controlling or domineering. Out of balance, a Pitta type can get quite angry and critical.

The attractive qualities of Pitta are their warm smile, penetrating gaze, vast knowledge on many subjects and their ability to reach and achieve goals.

Kapha Dosha

Kapha types are comprised of water (*jala*) and earth (*prithivi*).

Qualities of Kapha	When Balanced:	Out of Balance: Mind	Out of Balance: Body
Cool	Calm / patient	Greedy	Excess mucous/congestion
Heavy	Trustworthy	Possessive/ clingy	Weight gain
Slow	Faithful	Withdrawn	Expresses inertia
Wet/moist	Methodical/ careful about details	Depressed/ blue/ suffer from Seasonal Affective Disorder	Excess water/bloating/ swelling/ edema
Smooth	Affectionate / loving	Deep confusion	Overeating
Sweet	Great stamina	Hoarding	Lethargic
Dense	Smooth skin	Cravings	PMS

A Kapha person is endomorphic. Everything about their body structure is bigger and larger. The words for Kapha are *structure* and *stability*. Since Kapha is composed of the elements of water (*jala*) and earth (*prithivi*), it is a heavier dosha than the other two. Kapha types complain of being overweight.

Kaphas have a sweet personality. They are loving, kind, trustworthy, affectionate and forgiving. They are reliable and faithful. They learn slowly but have a great retentive memory. If you offend them, they will forgive you but they will never forget.

The body structure of a Kapha is solid. They have thick bountiful hair that is usually wavy. Their skin is soft and smooth.

A Kapha person's energy level is steady. They can sustain exercise and even lovemaking for a long time. But they do walk and move slow. They are methodical and careful.

When Kapha types get out of balance, they have a tendency toward inertia, holding in feelings, emotions, food, and tend to get depressed. An out-of-balance Kapha may be possessive with loved ones or begin to hoard material items. They may also be resistant to change.

Combining the doshas if you are a two-dosha type

Confusion in treating the doshas can come in if you are a two-dosha type or if your prakruti is combined. For most people, this is the case, since single dosha types are rare as are tri-doshic types.

As a general rule, you want to balance the most dominant dosha first. If you aren't too imbalanced, eating, exercising and using herbs for your dominant dosha should balance you rather quickly. However, if you are severely imbalanced or it's the season of your less-dominant dosha, balancing may start with a different dosha first. With disease, it often takes an experienced Ayurvedic practitioner to get you on the road to healing.

Below, I have given examples of two dosha types with symptoms and scenarios to demonstrate what might be done to regain balance.

The Pitta-Vata Type

A Pitta-Vata type might show traits of a Pitta mind and a Vata body or a combination of the two. An example might be someone who is medium in build, with a great appetite, intense, career oriented, driven and a perfectionist. But this person will also show traits of creativity, connection and communication with others and perhaps nervousness.

A person in this category would normally balance Pitta first, especially in spring, summer and perhaps early fall. In late fall and winter, it may be favorable to balance Vata.

Signs that Vata should be balanced first

Since Pitta is a hot dosha and it is also wet, a Pitta-Vata person who becomes, for example, cold, dry, nervous, and suffers from constipation, would indicate a Vata imbalance and therefore would need a Vata balancing program. The careful balancing act comes in, with a two-dosha type such as this, to not create an imbalance in the dominant dosha while balancing the second. The suggestion then, would be to eat a Vata pacifying diet for a few days to see if the symptoms subside.

The Vata-Kapha Type

Someone who is a Vata-Kapha typically has more traits of a Vata mind and a Kapha body or vice versa. My middle child is a Vata-Kapha and he is very thin with angular features, tall and fidgety when active. He paces when he talks on the phone to friends and eats fast. But his personality is laid-back and slow to accomplish tasks. He is compassionate, loving, kind and affectionate. He is quick to forgive and is a faithful friend. He likes to reflect before acting. He could sit on the couch for hours with a good book and it's sometimes hard to get him moving.

A Vata-Kapha would normally balance Vata first. But since these doshas are somewhat opposite, it's important to be careful and not bring the second dosha out of balance.

Signs that Kapha should be balanced first

A Vata-Kapha that shows signs of a Kapha imbalance may include excessive weight gain, water retention, inertia, congestion, allergies, or seasonal depression. In these cases or if other Kapha symptoms are present, balance Kapha first.

The Vikruti Test

Your *prakruti* is your genetic make up. It is your proportion of Vata, Pitta and Kapha in your mind and body. This was the genetic deck you were dealt with at the time of your conception and you cannot change it, nor would you want to. *Vikruti* means current state or state of imbalance. Through our experiences and choices, our doshas are in constant flux. Most of this is due to what we do and experience, but some of it is due to what's going on in the environment as nature affects our states as well. When you are feeling imbalanced, it's a good idea to take inventory of the doshas and where you might be feeling the imbalance. The Vikruti Test will help you make this assessment.

Instructions: When answering the prompts below, look back only to the past 60 days. Answering "0" means it does not apply to you and "5" means it applies almost all the time.

Section I: Vata

Lately I've been feeling anxious or worried.	0	1	2	3	4	5
I've been constipated or having a hard time moving my bowels.	0	1	2	3	4	5
My mind has been racing like crazy and it seems the thoughts never stop.	0	1	2	3	4	5
My skin or my eyes have been very dry.	0	1	2	3	4	5
My eating and sleeping patterns have become erratic.	0	1	2	3	4	5
My stomach has been feeling nervous or queasy.	0	1	2	3	4	5
I've been having a hard time going to sleep or have been awakening easily.	0	1	2	3	4	5
I'm forgetting things often.	0	1	2	3	4	5
I've been losing weight without trying.	0	1	2	3	4	5
I've been fearful or paranoid.	0	1	2	3	4	5

Section II: Pitta

I've been experiencing acid reflux or heartburn.	0	1	2	3	4	5
I've been experiencing loose stool.	0	1	2	3	4	5
I've been feeling critical and intolerant of others or myself.	0	1	2	3	4	5
I've been feeling hot or have been having hot flashes.	0	1	2	3	4	5
My skin has been breaking out in acne or rashes.	0	1	2	3	4	5
I've experienced more anger than usual.	0	1	2	3	4	5
I've been more impatient.	0	1	2	3	4	5
I've been overeating and I haven't felt good afterward.	0	1	2	3	4	5
I've been obsessed with finishing projects and making them perfect.	0	1	2	3	4	5
I've been overly competitive and concerned about winning.	0	1	2	3	4	5

Section III: Kapha

I've been craving sweets a lot and eating in between meals.	0	1	2	3	4	5
I've been oversleeping and taking naps.	0	1	2	3	4	5
I've been having a lot of congestion or sinus troubles.	0	1	2	3	4	5
I've been gaining weight.	0	1	2	3	4	5
I've been holding onto too many things in my house.	0	1	2	3	4	5
I've been feeling kind of blue lately or depressed.	0	1	2	3	4	5
Even though I've had some negative feelings about recent events, I have not wanted to deal with it.	0	1	2	3	4	5
I've been spending more time in front of the TV or computer and less time out exercising or doing activities.	0	1	2	3	4	5
I've lost my inner drive to try new things.	0	1	2	3	4	5
I've been recently diagnosed with diabetes, borderline diabetes, heart disease, or high blood pressure.	0	1	2	3	4	5

Score for Section I: Vata _____

Score for Section II: Pitta _____

Score for Section III: Kapha _____

Interpreting Your Vikruti Test

Your vikruti results are giving you a snapshot of where you are today in relation to your natural mind body constitution. Remember, these results can and will change from day to day or week to week. It all depends on your lifestyle and events going on currently in your life.

If your vikruti matches your prakruti you will know to balance your primary dosha first. In the event that your secondary dosha comes first in the Vikruti Test, you will balance that dosha first. In some cases, your third or least prominent dosha will show up on top in the Vikruti Test. Typically this shows great imbalance. It's important that you pay attention and work on rebalancing, not only to get your doshas back to where they need to be, but also learn to maintain balance on a daily basis to prevent disease from occurring.

Example: Let's suppose you are a Vata-Pitta type on your prakruti test in *The Wheel of Healing with Ayurveda* book. Remember, this is your true nature. You cannot change your prakruti. However, when you take the vikruti test in the *Companion Workbook*, your Pitta score is higher than your Vata score. In this case, you will balance Pitta first. Perhaps you've been experiencing skin rashes, acne and you've been more irritable than usual. Foods that normally don't bother you, are now giving you acid reflux or loose stool. These are all indications that Pitta is out of balance. For you to feel normal, your Pitta must return to a lower level. In order to achieve your balance, you can begin a Pitta pacifying diet, drink Pitta tea, take Pitta pacifying herbs, stay cool, immerse yourself in nature, do some emotional clearing and take time to meditate. You will continue your Pitta pacifying regime until you have a noticeable difference in your aggravated Pitta symptoms.

Exercise: Your Current Symptoms

After completing the Vikruti Test, make a list of your current symptoms. Notice if your symptoms match the dosha that was out of balance in your Vikruti Test.

_____
_____
_____
_____

Your Dosha Balancing Plan

The idea behind dosha balancing is to prevent the development of disease. Remember that in Ayurveda we try to detect imbalances before the full eruption of illness. Below are some suggestions to rebalance. Circle the ones you are willing to try.

I will try a dosha specific diet for my dosha that is out of balance.	I will try a vegetarian or vegan diet with the 12 Guidelines to an Ayurvedic Lifestyle diet as outlined in *The Wheel of Healing with Ayurveda*.	I will consult and take appropriate Ayurvedic herbs specific to a symptom or set of symptoms.	I will eliminate toxic substances such as alcohol, tobacco or drugs. (With guidance of an addiction specialist if needed.)
I will practice yoga daily.	I will start or continue a daily meditation practice.	I will create an Ayurvedic daily routine.	I will work on emotional clearing and healing my past.
I will work through the Routine for Optimal Sleep as outlined in *The Wheel of Healing with Ayurveda*.	Relationship healing. (With the guidance of a licensed therapist if needed.)	I will work on discovering my life's purpose.	I will spend more time in nature.
I will explore my spiritual life including my unique practice of religion or spiritual rituals and traditions.	I will create my list of intentions and desires.	I will limit time spent on electronic devices and increase my activity time.	I will make time for leisure activities such as hobbies, sports, creative outlets and friendships.
I will clear out my living and workspace of clutter.	I will heal my finances.	I will create a dosha specific exercise program.	I will explore a new career or job position if job dissatisfaction is an issue.
With my physician, I will work on lowering the number of prescription medications if possible.	I will find time to volunteer and give back by sharing my talents.	I will work on chakra clearing of blocked chakras.	

Now that you've selected the areas you are willing to work on to balance your doshas and your life, you can begin with the workbook chapter that most pertains to the strongest area of need.

CHAPTER TWO

A 15-DAY EXPLORATION *of* DHARMA

In order to begin your fifteen-day exploration of dharma, please read thoroughly the chapter on dharma in *The Wheel of Healing with Ayurveda*.

Often we move through life without purposeful direction. We acquire the material things needed to survive and perhaps, thrive. At the end of the day, we may wonder what this life is all about. Sometimes the thought may bring about discomfort and we push it away with alcohol, video games, a reality TV show or some other distraction. When we begin to question our purpose, this is a good time to entertain those thoughts, not push them out. The very essence of why we are here is to fulfill our mission we were created for. Finding that mission or purpose is the first step.

Day one: Watch, observe and jot down.
Today you are going to watch yourself as you go throughout the day. Notice what makes you happy, joyful and thankful. Which activities are you enjoying? Which activities don't you enjoy? Who do you like to spend time with? What do those people bring to you as gifts? How do you make others laugh or smile? If there is little to no joy, look inside to see what is bothering you. Don't make any judgments; just write down these observations today.

My observations for today:
_____
_____
_____
_____
_____

Day two: What is your driving force?
Driving force is big. Today, notice what motivates you. What makes you get out of bed in the morning? Do you have the drive to jump out of bed and seize the day? Or does getting out of bed make you moan and groan? As you go throughout your day, what drives you to perform? Love, commitment, passion, money, security, service? Whatever you notice, write it down.

My driving forces:
_____
_____
_____
_____
_____

Day three: What are your natural talents?
Natural talents are things you are good at without even trying. It's almost as if you don't understand how you know how to do something, it just flows easily. An example might be playing the piano by ear, even though you've never had a lesson. Another example might be creating successful companies, even though you have no business background or a business degree. Your natural talents are important to understand because often, these lead us to our life's purpose.

My Natural Talents:
_____
_____
_____
_____
_____

Day four: What are your passions?
Passions are things that you love and you love to do but aren't necessarily naturally talented at. These things require a little more work for you. It may take some lessons or learning to hone the skills of your passions. For example, you love to paint but painting doesn't come naturally for you. Yet, you are willing to join a painting class to learn all you can and improve your skill. Another example is a passion for cooking. Perhaps cooking gives you great joy but you need to follow recipes or the food doesn't turn out that great. However, when you watch the Cooking Channel and learn new tricks and tips, you see your cooking improve each time.

My Passions:
_____
_____
_____
_____
_____

Day five: Which of your natural talents or passions do you practice weekly?
It's important that you reflect on this. Even if, at first glance, it may seem that you don't practice very many of them each week, you may see more of your talents and passions come out in subtle ways. For example, let's say you are a mother who is passionate about breastfeeding for babies. You may no longer have a baby at home, who is breastfeeding, but you notice that each time you see a pregnant woman, you engage in a conversation with her about the benefits of breastfeeding. While that is not a weekly practice, it is a frequent practice that shows up on a casual basis.

I practice these natural talents and passions weekly:
_____
_____
_____
_____
_____

Day six: My retirement dream
Often, we hear people say, "When I retire, I'm going to..." This may be an indication of your dharma or your life's purpose if this is something you also say. If you were going to retire tomorrow, what would you do? How would you go about doing it?

When I retire I would like to...
_____
_____
_____
_____
_____

Day seven: What do I waste my time on?
We all do it, procrastination and time wasting. We are creatures of habit and often repeat the same things day after day. Observe yourself today and notice how you waste time. Do you constantly surf the Internet, text people silly pictures, spend too much time on Facebook, or search for things in piles of clutter? Maybe your TV is always on and you spend too much time watching it.

There is a difference between "down time" or unwinding time and wasted time or procrastination. Often we may see ourselves wasting time because we are tired, don't want to deal with emotions or a situation or using it as avoidance for something we need to do.

I often waste my time on:
_____
_____
_____
_____

Day Eight: A Journey Down Memory Lane
When you were young, what did you dream of becoming? What did you tell others you would study or choose as a career? Was there a career that fascinated you in particular as a child? Write down anything that comes to mind as you scan your childhood for ideas.

As a child, I often thought about becoming a/an...
_____
_____

_____
_____
_____

Day Nine: If I could do this, I wouldn't consider it work.
Looking over all of your answers above, think about what you could be doing, for many hours per day, and it wouldn't seem like work for you. If you did this one thing, you would jump out of bed, early in the morning with enthusiasm. At night, you would almost not want to go to sleep because that would mean stopping this activity. Thinking about doing this activity makes you blissful.

My one activity I could do all day long:
_____
_____
_____
_____
_____

Day Ten: A Career, A Second Job, or an Extended Hobby
Living your dharma or purpose in life doesn't always mean that your purpose is embedded as a career choice. Often, it's more convenient when the two match because, after all, it would be better to earn an income while living our your life's purpose. But that is not always the case. As you think about this one activity that has your heart, imagine if you can create a career out of it. If that doesn't seem feasible now, imagine when it could happen. Would it be possible to do your beloved activity as a second job, such as in the evenings or on weekends? Or would it be possible to have it as an extended hobby during much of your free time? Look back to day seven and notice how much time you can save if you let go of some of the time wasting activities. You could replace those with your blissful activity. Right now, don't worry about cost, training or education. That will come later. Focus on how you can make this possible and under what capacity you can make your dream come true.

My one blissful activity can become a career, a second job or an extended hobby in this way:
_____
_____
_____
_____
_____

Day Eleven: Preparation to live my dharma
Now that you've decided under what capacity you will live out your dream activity, explore your preparedness to begin. Let's suppose, you're a medical doctor, but your dream is to teach surfing lessons. You may have never been trained to teach surfing. What would it take to get you to a point where you could do that? What certifications might you need? Would you have to relocate? Or perhaps you'd like to run a home day care and you've been an administrative assistant for ten years. What courses in child development would you have to consider? What licenses and certifications would you need to run a childcare in your home? Look for other people who do what you'd like to be doing. Browse their websites and visit their places of business. Do not assess cost yet. Just gather information.

I've found that I need these things to be able to begin living my dharma:
_____
_____
_____
_____
_____

Day Twelve: Assessing Costs and Creative Solutions to Living my Dharma
Unless your blissful activity is pure volunteerism, there are usually costs associated with living your dharma. Even if you are contemplating running a non-profit, there are still costs involved. When doing your day eleven activity, you may have noticed that you need certain licenses or certifications. Maybe you even need a degree. Or perhaps you need start up costs for a business. Know, that there are many different ways to live your dharma at any income level. You will need to get creative at this point. If you need training, you can offer to be an apprentice under someone who is already working in your field. For example, I am happy to train yoga teachers as interns at my studio if it means they will stay and teach for me. Many times you can volunteer your way into organizations. There are loans, grants and scholarships for many different fields of study. If you're starting your own small business, there are many things you can do yourself at a very low cost. Visit your local Chamber of Commerce or starting going to business networking groups and ask people for pointers. You can avoid costly mistakes by getting great advice from people who have started small businesses or non-profits.

These are the costs I may face when beginning to live my dharma:
_____
_____

Day Thirteen: These Things Could Possibly Hold Me Back & Solutions

In any endeavor, there are always things that may hold you back. To live your dharma is no different. If there weren't things holding you back, you would be living your blissful activity now. Think of possible things, people, situations or circumstances that may stop you from living your dharma. Then, think of solutions to allow you to move forward. Do not leave this activity until you have thought of a solution to every possible hold back.

These things may hold me back and here are the solutions:

_____
_____
_____
_____
_____

Day Fourteen: Moving Forward with my Dharma

Today you will do something that moves you toward your life's purpose. It could be making a phone call, sending an email or purchasing a book. You can also create a visual board with images, quotes or anything else that will help you move toward living your dream. What we focus on, we move toward. Keep reminders of where you'd like to be in a month, six months and a year out in front of you. Post it on your bathroom mirror. Leave it on your nightstand or keep an image on your computer. Remind yourself constantly so you never forget your bliss and make it a reality.

Things I will do today to help me move toward my dharma:

_____
_____
_____
_____
_____

Day Fifteen: Tell at least two people you trust about your blissful activity and your plans to make it real.

Words have power. And when you say things aloud, you are speaking them into existence. Even if you are still feeling skeptical about whether or not you can make your dreams a reality, speak as though it is already happening. Speak with confidence and conviction. You've already worked through your possible obstacles and the solutions to overcoming them, so you have nothing to fear. Choose two people you trust completely and also those who are less likely to judge or question you. Tell them your plans. Ask them if they will support you in your endeavor. Friends and family who believe in you will support you in any way they can, even if it's just being your cheerleader.

I can tell these two people in my life about my dharma and here's why:
_____
_____
_____
_____
_____

Your journey to living your dharma does not end here. Make sure you set mini-goals and intentions to accomplish at least one task every day to move you toward your dharma. Write down your intentions and read them before you meditate each day. Visualize yourself doing exactly what you were created to do and begin living the life of your dreams.

CHAPTER THREE

PHYSICAL HEALTH PART ONE: DOSHA SPECIFIC DIETS

A good way to begin healing and to alleviate symptoms is to focus on a dosha specific diet. Before you begin your dosha regime, make sure you have shifted your eating habits to include the *12 Guidelines for an Ayurvedic Lifestyle Eating Plan* as outlined on page 58 in *The Wheel of Healing with Ayurveda*. Once you have added these principles to your lifestyle, you are ready to start the diet; which will pacify your aggravated dosha.

To recap, remember that each of the doshas is comprised of two of the great elements from the *mahabhutas:* space, air, fire, water and earth. When a dosha is aggravated, one or both of these elements are too high in your mind and body. For example, if you are a Kapha type, your primary elements are water and earth. If the Kapha dosha is out of balance, that means you have too much water and/or earth in your mind-body constitution. Keep in mind that you do not need more of what you already have. In this example, you already have a fair amount of water and earth. Therefore, you do not need more of it. When you begin your Kapha-pacifying diet, you will be lowering the amount of water and earth so your Kapha symptoms will subside.

Even while balancing, you need to keep in mind that you will need to get all six tastes at every meal. In a dosha balancing diet, however, you will eat more of the tastes that will pacify your dosha and less of the tastes which may aggravate your dosha. If it seems complicated now, once you begin reading over the dosha plans and applying them to your life, it will become easier.

The Vata Pacifying Diet: Promote Calm and Serenity

Increase: Sweet, Sour and Salty
Decrease: Bitter, Pungent and Astringent

The elements of space and air make up a Vata type. When Vata is aggravated, these elements are more present in a person's mind and body. The sweet, sour and salty tastes will help lower the amount of space and air. Include smaller amounts, however, of the bitter, pungent and astringent tastes. Generally speaking, you will portion your plate as follows: 75% sweet, sour and salty and the other 25% bitter, pungent and astringent. On page 64 and 65 of *The Wheel of Healing with Ayurveda*, you will find foods lists with each of the six tastes. I must emphasize that the sweet taste includes most foods that are naturally sweet or have a baseline taste of sweet. All too often, it's easy to get carried away and interpret eating sweet as filling with cake, cookies and muffins. When in reality, the sweet taste is perceived by sweet fruit, rice, pasta, meat, chicken and oils. Also, it's easy to add too much salt. A little salt goes a long way.

An example of a balanced Vata breakfast would be a whole grain Cream of Wheat or Cream of Rice (sweet & astringent) made with 2% organic grass-fed milk (sweet) and sweetened with maple syrup (sweet), cinnamon, and nutmeg (sweet and pungent). You could add a side of orange juice (sour) or grapefruit sections (sour). And for a beverage a black coffee or black tea with a dash of cardamom would add the bitter taste. If you add a dash of salt to the hot cereal, you will have all six tastes represented.

As you can see, it is fairly easy to integrate all six tastes in a meal. In the beginning, it will require some focus and attention but in a short time, it will become second nature. Look over the Six Tastes List in *The Wheel of Healing with Ayurveda* and jot down foods you naturally enjoy in the sweet, sour and salty categories.

Sweet	Sour	Salty

Key Points to Keep in Mind When Preparing a Vata Meal

1. Increase the sweet, sour and salty tastes.

2. Decrease the bitter, pungent and astringent tastes.

3. Eat warm or hot food and decrease cold or iced foods and beverages.

4. Drink warm water or herbal tea during mealtime.

5. Cook with fats such as butter, ghee, olive oil or canola oil.

6. Choose sautéing and boiling over baking or grilling.

7. Opt for dairy products which are 2% or greater in fat content.

8. Eat in a settled environment without too much stimuli.

9. Use warming and sweet spices such as cardamom, nutmeg, and cinnamon.

10. Try Vata pacifying teas and spice mixes.

11. Minimize dry foods such as crackers, rice cakes, nuts and dried fruit.

Create Your Own Vata Meal Plan

Using the knowledge in *The Wheel of Healing with Ayurveda* and the explanations above, create your Vata pacifying meal plan with two options for each meal including snacks. In parentheses next to the foods, you will list the taste of each food. Many foods have more than one taste but most have a main taste and secondary or tertiary tastes.

Breakfast
#1 _____
_____
_____
_____
_____
#2 _____
_____
_____
_____
_____

Lunch
#1 _____
_____
_____
_____
#2 _____
_____

Dinner
#1 _____

#2 _____

Snacks
_____

The Pitta Pacifying Diet: Remain Cool and Calm

Increase: Sweet, Bitter and Astringent
Decrease: Sour, Salty and Pungent

Do you know the expression "cool as a cucumber"? That is exactly the idea with a Pitta pacifying diet. In fact, cucumbers are one of the cooling foods for Pitta. Comprised of the elements of fire and water, Pitta types tend to be warm and moist. When the fire gets too high, they are hot, irritable, cranky and critical. Their bodies' sweat and their skin become red.

To pacify Pitta, you must lower the heat and at times reduce the amount of water in the body. On a plate, you will have 75% of the sweet, bitter and astringent tastes and only 25% of the sour, salty and pungent tastes. Pitta types must be careful about overeating, eating fried food and drinking alcohol. Ayurveda considers alcohol to be *tamasic* (low energy) and in most cases should not be consumed. Pitta types are especially sensitive to the effects of alcohol.

Since a Pitta person has strong *agni* (digestive fire), it is easy for him or her to eat too much and gain weight. While meat is not bad for a Pitta, it is a heating food and in general, Pitta types do much better with a vegetarian diet.

An example of a Pitta dinner might be a fresh water fish grilled (sweet), topped with a mango chutney (sweet), with grilled asparagus (bitter & astringent) and a fresh spinach salad (bitter & astringent) with sliced almonds (sweet & bitter), strawberries (sweet & sour), vinegar (sour) and olive oil (sweet). By adding salt and pepper to your fish or salad, you will have added both the salty and pungent tastes but not in excess.

Now, look over the Six Tastes List in *The Wheel of Healing with Ayurveda* and jot down foods you naturally enjoy in the sweet, bitter and astringent categories.

Sweet	Bitter	Astringent

Key Points to Keep in Mind When Preparing a Pitta Meal

1. Increase sweet, bitter and astringent.

2. Decrease sour, salty and pungent.

3. Strive for cooling foods such as cucumbers, mint, melons, ripe mangoes, cilantro, sweet ripened pears, plums and cherries.

4. Avoid fried foods, spicy food and alcoholic beverages.

5. Replace red meat with fresh water fish and white poultry or go vegetarian.

6. Pay attention to the *Ten Guidelines for Eating Awareness* on page 71 of *The Wheel of Healing with Ayurveda*.

7. Eliminate iced beverages.

8. Try Pitta pacifying teas and spice mixes.

9. Choose grilling or baking as methods of cooking over sautéing and boiling.

10. Eat on a schedule so you can catch the body while it's hungry but no too deprived. Besides getting cranky, you may find you overeat when your hunger is out of control.

Create Your Own Pitta Meal Plan

Using the knowledge in *The Wheel of Healing with Ayurveda* and the explanations above, create your Pitta pacifying meal plan with two options for each meal including snacks. In parentheses next to the foods, you will list the taste of each food. Many foods have more than one taste but most have a main taste and secondary or tertiary tastes.

Breakfast
#1 _____
_____

#2 _____

Lunch
#1 _____

#2 _____

Dinner
#1 _____

#2 _____

Snacks

Kapha Pacifying Diet for Weight Loss

Increase: Bitter, Pungent and Astringent
Decrease: Sweet, Sour and Salty

Kapha types may find they are constantly struggling with body weight. Comprised of the elements of water and earth, Kapha people naturally find themselves on the heavier side and being that their metabolism and digestion are slower, it is also difficult for them to lose weight.

If you are a Kapha type, it may be difficult for you to overcome inertia when your Kapha is out of balance. You may not want to exercise and you may crave sweet foods such as ice cream, cookies and cake. But with your stamina and endurance, you can celebrate a long, healthy life if you keep your Kapha balanced without excess weight.

Kapha types will fill their plate with 75% of the bitter, pungent and astringent tastes and 25% percent with the sweet, sour and salty tastes. A Kapha must be careful about snacking and stick to mealtimes for eating. In fact, according to Ayurveda, a Kapha can get by with two complete meals per day. Even if you decide to plan three meals in the day, try to eat the first meal closer to 9:30 or 10 a.m. and make sure you eat the last meal by 6:30 p.m. In order to lose weight with a Kapha pacifying diet, you want to make sure you do not snack in between meals. Also, it a great idea to pay attention to portion sizes.

A complete Kapha pacifying meal may look like this: a Greek style salad made Romaine lettuce (astringent), cucumbers (sweet & astringent), grape tomatoes (sweet & sour), bell peppers (sweet & astringent), 6 Kalamata olives (bitter & sweet), 2 TB of feta cheese (sour & salty), 1/4 cup garbanzo beans (astringent), 1 TB of each: fresh dill (astringent), cilantro (astringent & sweet), parsley (astringent & pungent). Add a dressing of 2TB of fresh lemon juice (sour), 2 tsp of olive oil (sweet), 1 garlic clove (pungent), crushed salt (salty) and pepper (pungent) to taste. To complete the meal, you can add a slice of whole-wheat pita bread (sweet & astringent) and a ¼ cup of homemade hummus (astringent, pungent, sour, sweet, and salty).

Now, look over the Six Tastes List in *The Wheel of Healing with Ayurveda* and jot down foods you naturally enjoy in the bitter, pungent and astringent categories.

Bitter	Pungent	Astringent

Key Points to Keep in Mind When Preparing a Kapha Meal

1. Increase the bitter, pungent and astringent tastes.

2. Decrease the sweet, sour and salty tastes.

3. Reduce dairy, which increases Kapha in the body.

4. Favor beans, lentils, fish and chicken and reduce meat eating only once or twice per month.

5. Eat a salad at every meal after breakfast.

6. Eliminate fried foods.

7. Eat warm, light foods (not too much butter or oil).

8. Increase raw fruits and vegetables.

9. Eat a light breakfast during late Kapha period: 9-10 a.m.

10. Add spice to stimulate weight loss and increase metabolism. Examples are cardamom, cinnamon, coriander, cumin, fennel, garam masala, and ginger. (Cumin, fenugreek, sesame seed, and turmeric are both bitter and astringent.)

10. Drink warm water throughout the day.

11. Favor dry cooking methods such as: baking, broiling, grilling, sautéing rather than steaming, boiling, poaching which can increase water in the body.

12. Stimulate the appetite by taking a bitter or pungent taste at the beginning of the meal rather than salty or sour. Examples: Eat Romaine lettuce or endive (bitter) or fresh ginger root (pungent).

13. To stave off hunger drink one of the two following teas: Hot water, 1 TB of fresh lime juice, 1 tsp of honey or hot ginger tea: 1 TB of freshly minced ginger, 1 tsp of honey, 1 TB of fresh lemon juice. These teas increase metabolism, scrape the fat out of the channels in the body, and reduce hunger.

15. Try Kapha pacifying teas and spice mixes.

16. Eat a light dinner no later than 6:30 p.m.

17. Avoid eating 3 hours prior to bedtime.

Create Your Own Kapha Meal Plan

Using the knowledge in *The Wheel of Healing with Ayurveda* and the explanations above, create your Kapha pacifying meal plan with two options for each meal. In this section, I have not included lines for snacks since the goal is to stick with 2-3 meals in a day. In parentheses next to the foods, you will list the taste of each food. Many foods have more than one taste but most have a main taste and secondary or tertiary tastes.

Breakfast
#1 _____
_____
_____
_____
_____

#2 _____
_____
_____
_____
_____
_____

Lunch
#1 _____
_____
_____
_____
_____

#2 _____
_____
_____
_____
_____
_____

Dinner
#1 _____
_____
_____
_____

#2 _____
_____
_____
_____
_____

Weight Loss for All the Doshas

Weight gain is not limited to a person with a Kapha dominant mind body type. Vata and Pitta types can and do also gain weight. The question I most often get is if it is O.K. to follow a Kapha pacifying diet when a person's dominant dosha is not Kapha. The answer is to proceed with caution. A Vata type who begins a Kapha diet to lose weight is eating a larger portion of the three tastes, which he must naturally reduce. If he stays on this diet too long, he will find a rapid increase of the space and air qualities, which, in turn, will bring a whole host of undesired symptoms. The same goes for a Pitta type. While a Pitta and a Kapha diet are not too different. The difference is in the minimal amount of sweet on a Kapha diet and the inclusion of the pungent taste to increase metabolism. I have had Pitta clients on Kapha diets that have developed severe heartburn due to the increase in Kapha spices and the heat in Kapha-like foods.

So what then is the solution? If you are a dominant Vata or Pitta type who needs to lose weight, you may try a Kapha diet for a few days and notice how it affects your body. Another solution is to pay close attention to portion size and calorie count, even if you are eating for your own dosha. I have found that MyFitnessPal is a great, free application that helps you track your food intake. Coupled with a dosha appropriate exercise program, you can lose weight gently without going out of balance. Remember, in any weight loss regime, it's more about permanent lifestyle change, than about the method to weight loss.

CHAPTER FOUR

PHYSICAL HEALTH PART TWO: DAILY ROUTINE *and* EXERCISE

An Ayurvedic daily routine is a big part of lifestyle change and discipline. According to Ayurveda, there are optimal times to perform certain tasks. If we are to flow with the rhythms of nature, we can catch the waves of activity and rest that will help us move with our natural cycles rather than fight against them. Look at the twenty-four hour circadian clock according to the doshas on page 81 in *The Wheel of Healing with Ayurveda.* You will notice that the day is divided into six parts as each dosha governs a four-hour window twice daily.

As you adapt to your new lifestyle, you will need to fit new practices into your day. At first, it may seem overwhelming and nearly impossible. But I assure you that many people, with very busy lives, have been successful in including new Ayurvedic practices into their day. You may need to be creative but anything is possible if you want it. For example, I have suggested to clients that they use driving time to practice yoga breathing techniques, visualization, and mantra mini-meditations (with eyes open of course). Work lunch hours have become meditation time or walking time.

Here are some practices you may need to add to your daily routine:

Meditation
Yoga
Cardiovascular exercise
Strength training
Cooking fresh food/ food preparation
Yogic breathing techniques
Mealtimes with family or sitting for meals
Spending time outdoors or in nature
Creative expression time
Playtime
Optimal sleep time

Living a balanced life is not simply about working, eating and sleeping. It's about including many of the aspects you might often forget to maintain health, happiness and balance. When planning your Ayurvedic daily routine, you want to take into account exercising thirty to sixty minutes per day and varying the routine to include yoga or stretching, cardiovascular and strength training exercises. Below, we will explore the different activities for each of the doshas. The amount of sleep you need will vary on your mind body type. Vata types need about seven to eight hours of sleep. Pitta types can often get by with four to six hours. And Kapha types typically need between eight and ten hours of sleep. The general rule for all mind body types is to wake up before the first Kapha time occurs (around 8 a.m.) and it's often best to catch the hyper-metabolic state of Vata between 6 and 7 a.m. to feel the most alert for your day. Meditation is best done at sunrise and sunset. But I always teach my clients to fit meditation in whenever they can. Find pockets in the day to sneak in a meditation time.

My Ayurvedic Daily Routine

Take some time now and fill out your Ayurvedic daily routine.

6 a.m. _____
6:30 a.m. _____
7 a.m. _____
7:30 a.m. _____
8 a.m. _____
8:30 a.m. _____
9 a.m. _____
9:30 a.m. _____
10 a.m. _____
10:30 a.m. _____
11 a.m. _____
11:30 a.m. _____
12 p.m. _____
12:30 p.m. _____
1 p.m. _____
1:30 p.m. _____
2 p.m. _____
2:30 p.m. _____
3 p.m. _____
3:30 p.m. _____
4 p.m. _____
4:30 p.m. _____
5 p.m. _____
5:30 p.m. _____
6 p.m. _____
6:30 p.m. _____
7 p.m. _____
7:30 p.m. _____
8 p.m. _____
8:30 p.m. _____
9 p.m. _____
9:30 p.m. _____
10 p.m. _____
10:30 p.m. _____
11 p.m. _____

According to Ayurveda, you should be asleep between the hours of 11 p.m. (at the latest) and 5:30 a.m. to allow your body time to rest, rejuvenate, detoxify and clear the mind. Your before bed routine should begin between 10 and 10:30 p.m.

Daily Exercise

Moving your body is important for physical, mental and emotional wellbeing. Ideally, the activities you choose should also be pleasurable. If you are not taking pleasure in your exercise program, you may be creating toxins in the body instead of healing chemicals. The sky is the limit when it comes to physical activity. As mentioned in *The Wheel of Healing with Ayurveda,* there are certain parameters when it comes to moving for your mind body type. Kaphas need vigorous activity for a longer duration. Pitta types need less competitive activity and need to stay cool. Vata types need to vary activity and opt for gentle movement. Explore the activities below and circle the ones that seem more appealing to you.

Brisk Walking	Tai Chi	Skating	Swimming	Working out in a gym	Elliptical machine
Hatha Yoga	Qi Gong	Skiing	Soccer	Working out outdoors	Rowing machine
Hot Yoga	Karate	Running or jogging	Tennis	Gardening/ Lawn mowing	Bike riding/ cycling
Vinyasa Flow Yoga	Step Aerobics	Weight lifting	Triathalons	Football	Body resistance training (push ups, sit ups etc.)
Dance	Zumba	Snorkeling or scuba diving	Golf	Volleyball	Hiking
Rock climbing	Stair climbing	Baseball or softball	Basketball	Kickboxing	Pilates

Physical Health Part Two: Daily Routine and Exercise

Strive to plan an activity for each day of the week, even if it's a 20-30 minute brisk walk. Integrate the three components of a complete exercise program on a weekly basis: cardiovascular, strength training and stretching.

My Exercise Plan

Monday: _____

Tuesday: _____

Wednesday: _____

Thursday: _____

Friday: _____

Saturday: _____

Sunday: _____

CHAPTER FIVE

PHYSICAL HEALTH PART THREE: DETOXIFICATION *of* the BODY

Gentle detoxification of the body is an integral part of practicing an Ayurvedic lifestyle. We are constantly accumulating toxins and the body is an amazing filtration system that seamlessly removes most of them. However, since our nutrition is not always optimal and because there are environmental factors we cannot control, we do accumulate toxins that we need to consciously work on removing to stay at optimal levels of health. The word for toxins in Ayurveda is *ama*, which translates to toxic residue or a sticky substance that remains in the circulatory channels of the body. We can either remove ama gently on a daily basis or on a monthly or seasonal basis. Below are some exercises you can try to detoxify the body.

Exercise 1: Prepare Your Body for Detoxification
When you begin to eat an Ayurvedic lifestyle diet, you are already gently detoxifying your body. Follow The Twelve Guidelines for an Ayurvedic Lifestyle Eating Plan in *The Wheel of Healing with Ayurveda*. In addition, you can go on a kitchen detox. Look through your cupboards and remove and throw away all packaged food with artificial flavorings or colors, hydrogenated oils, MSG, white, enriched flour, corn syrup, artificial sweeteners, and expired products. Go through your fridge and do the same. Also, throw away prepared food that is more than 24-hours old. This includes food, you may have prepared and stored in the freezer. As for beverages, aim to drink only fresh juice, water, herbal tea, black or green tea and coffee (in small quantities). Warm milk is acceptable, according to Ayurveda, but is considered a complete meal and therefore, should be consumed separately from other meals. Avoid drinking alcohol, soda and other sugar-laden beverages.

Exercise 2: Gentle Ayurvedic Practices: Tongue Scraping, Hot Water Therapy, Herbal Oil Massage.
Once you've completed and implemented the first exercise, you are ready to begin integrating some gentle Ayurvedic detoxification practices. Each morning after brushing your teeth, use a tongue scraper to gently clean your tongue. Toxins accumulate on the tongue during sleep and tongue scraping helps remove them and freshens your breath. It also helps to stimulate the gastro-colic reflex, which helps you feel the urge to move your bowels, an added bonus. There are different types of tongue scrapers available but I've found that a stainless steel one works best.

Hot water therapy works wonders to get your body to remove toxins. Throughout the day, take small sips of hot water (at the temperature you would use for hot tea) frequently. The amount of water is less important than the frequency. You can also add a little honey to taste. Honey itself can help to scrape fat from the circulatory channels in the body. If you are diabetic, skip the honey. Make sure the water is very hot and drink from morning until night.

Ayurvedic self-administered massage is called *abhyanga*. The skin is the largest organ in the body, making up 10% of your body weight. Massaging an herbalized oil into the skin is an effective way to remove toxins and stimulate growth hormones. There are different oils for Vata, Pitta and Kapha. Each of these oils will have the proper herbs to balance your dosha. Before showering, you can heat up three to four tablespoons of the oil and place a towel on the bathroom floor. Gently rub the oil into your skin using up and down strokes on the extremities and circular motions on the joints, stomach and scalp. Get into the shower carefully (because you will be slippery) and allow the steam to open the pores and the oil will infuse into your body. If you choose, you can simply rinse off or use a gentle soap that will leave a light film of the herbal oil on your skin throughout the day.

Exercise 3: Simplify your eating and detoxify the colon.
As you are beginning to loosen ama in the body, you want to be able to remove it promptly. Taking a tablespoon of ground flaxseed three times daily can help to move your bowels more frequently. You can add the flaxseed to a cereal, yogurt, salad or any other dish. Flaxseed, that is fresh, has a nice nutty taste. It does go rancid rather quickly so keep it in the fridge and pay attention to the expiration date. Another method you can use is an Ayurvedic formula called *triphala*. Triphala is comprised of three Ayurvedic herbs: *amalaki*, *bibitaki* and *haritaki*. This formula is good for all three doshas. It helps rejuvenate cells and has a slight laxative effect that is not habit forming. If you are a Pitta type, it may aggravate your bowels a little too much. If this is the case, stop taking it or take it every other day. Take triphala in the evening, before bed, with a large glass of warm water. In the morning you will notice a more regular bowel movement. Several companies sell triphala in a tablet form. My favorite is sold through Banyan Botanicals. Start with one tablet at night and you can increase it to two after a few days.

If you wish to simplify your eating for a week, you can opt to eat rice, lentils and vegetables. There is an Ayurvedic recipe called *kitchari* and includes basmati rice, mung dal and spices such as turmeric, cumin, mustard seed, ginger and asafoetida. You can eat kitchari as a simple diet. For snack you can eat fresh fruit and drink fresh fruit juice. If your blood sugar tends to be high or you are diabetic, you can replace the rice with quinoa, which has a lower glycemic index. Many Americans don't have a habit of eating lentils. In that case, you can keep a simple vegetarian diet for the week. Try to stay away from processed sugar and convenience foods during this week. When you are able, replace coffee with an Ayurvedic dosha-specific tea. Another homemade detoxifying tea can be made with chopped fresh ginger, fresh lemon, honey and hot water. You can drink this throughout the day.

Exercise 4: Rejuvenate Your Cells
Once you've worked through detoxifying your body, you can begin to rejuvenate your cells. Continuing with an Ayurvedic lifestyle diet and exercise program, you can add rejuvenating herbs. An Ayurvedic herbal formula called *chaywanprash* has been around for thousands of years and is comprised of many Ayurvedic herbs but the main three ingredients are amla berry, ghee and honey. Amla berry or amalaki is revered as one of the most healing foods in Ayurveda. It has five of the six tastes and has nearly twenty times the amount of vitamin C than orange juice. Depending on the chaywanprash formula, it contains between twenty and eighty herbs. Studies have shown that taking

chaywanprash, while undergoing chemotherapy treatments, lowers the number of side effects in patients. In India, many families take this herbal jam like Americans take a multivitamin. The Himalayan Institute makes my favorite chaywanprash formula.

There are other Ayurvedic herbs that also work toward rejuvenating cells. In Sanskrit these are called *rasayanas.* If you're interested in integrating other herbs into your regime, it's best to consult with an Ayurvedic practitioner to see which ones are best for you.

Panchakarma and Ayurvedic Fasting

As I mentioned, detoxification of the body is a big part of Ayurveda. There is a special set of treatments in Ayurveda called *panchakarma.* The word panchakarma means "five actions" since there are five different steps toward cleansing. Some of these therapies include sweat therapy, warm oil massage, and herbal enemas. Panchakarma is best done under the supervision of an Ayurvedic practitioner or a center, which specializes in these cleansing practices.

Since Ayurveda teaches you to be gentle on the body, complete fasting is not recommended. Each dosha will fast in a different way. Vata types should only fast once per season and ideally at the changing of the seasons. As a Vata, you will eat fruit; drink fruit juices and vegetable broths. If you become too hungry, you can eat a simple meal of lentils and rice. Pitta types can try fasting once per month or every two months. Pittas can get by on fruit and vegetable juices. Kapha types can fast more often, even once weekly. During a Kapha fast, you can drink clear liquids and broths throughout the day. In any case, keep your fast to a 24-hour period.

CHAPTER SIX

SPIRITUAL HEALTH: CONNECTING DAILY

Living in touch with your spiritual-self daily is one of the key ways to remaining in balance. Our minds don't often know what it is we really want. What goes on in our minds tends to change with our mood or time of the day. Our egos know even less what we truly want. The ego is absorbed with instant gratification or doesn't take into account our higher purpose. Living in ego-consciousness often leads us astray and alienates us from others. The ego lives from a place of, "What's yours is mine and what's mine is mine." Yet, being able to live from our spiritual essence leads us closer to living in harmony; not only with ourselves, but with all of those around us.

As mentioned in *The Wheel of Healing with Ayurveda,* meditation is one of the best ways to get in touch with your spiritual self. Meditation allows you time to get quiet, lower the number of thoughts and begin exploration of the universe within. With few exceptions, most everyone can do meditation. My recommendation is to learn and do a mantra-based meditation technique such as the Chopra Center's Primordial Sound Meditation or Transcendental Meditation. But there are many different meditation techniques. If you have a prayer practice, you can add some meditation. I have heard this phrase, "Prayer is you talking to God. And meditation is allowing God to talk to you." I would have to agree. While I do have a daily prayer practice, I find that my meditation practice allows me to receive instead of give. Remember that meditation in itself is non-religious. There are certainly ways to make it religious but I am encouraging a practice of allowing you to open up to your higher self.

Exercise: Finding a meditation practice that works for you. Take some time and do research on finding a meditation practice that you can fit into your daily routine. Ideally, you will be meditating twice per day. A mantra-based practice recommends twenty to thirty minutes of meditation twice per day. Other practices will have varying times of meditation. You will need to allow time for your mind to settle into your practice, so anything less than fifteen minutes per session is usually not effective. Next, fill in the log and track your meditation times. I recommend picking one type of practice and sticking with it until it sticks with you. It will take about ninety days of consistent practice for you to form a healthy habit.

Types of meditation I have tried:

_____
_____
_____
_____
_____

I prefer these types of meditation:

_____
_____
_____
_____
_____

Spiritual Health: Connecting Daily

My meditation log:

Date/Time	Duration	Place	Experiences if any

Living a Spiritual Life Daily

You can take the following exercises and practice one weekly or once per day or mix it up. The more you open yourself to these practices, the more you will find your spiritual self expand.

1. **Practicing gratitude**
   Take some time and fill out the exercise on gratitude in the Introduction. Now list five things for which you can be grateful for each day.
   _____
   _____
   _____
   _____
   _____

2. **Have a namasté day**
   Notice what happens on the day you choose to honor each and every person you meet from the space of the heart and soul. When you took time today to silently bid each person *namasté,* how did you interactions change?
   _____
   _____
   _____
   _____
   _____
   _____

3. **Immerse yourself in nature.**
   Name three ways you will connect with nature this week:
   _____
   _____
   _____
   _____
   _____

4. **Embrace wonder and awe.**
   Today, observe the little things that make you say, "Wow!" Write them down.
   _____
   _____
   _____

5. **Take time to laugh each day.**
Laughter is the best medicine. Even if laughing doesn't come naturally for you, write down ways in which you can create genuine laughter (but not at another's expense, of course). Think of a funny show you like to watch or talk to a humorous friend. Maybe you share an inside joke with your spouse or partner. Write down three ways to incorporate laughter into your day.

6. **Give someone your full attention each day.**
This is a gift you can give someone for free. You can also give this gift to yourself. Not long ago, there was a study done in which children were asked to choose between an expensive gift and exclusive time with one of their parents. Every time the children chose exclusive parent time over the gift. In what ways can you give someone your full attention? How can you show him or her your attention is real and present?

7. **Hug often and touch often.**
Giving and receiving affection is a fundamental human need. Who do you hug every day? Who can you hug? Do you need to schedule in affection time with your significant other or your children? If so, do it now.

8. **Do random acts of kindness.**
   List at least five acts of kindness you can do this week. Remember, these are things for which you expect nothing in return.
   _____
   _____
   _____
   _____
   _____

9. **Forgive, let go, and move on.**
   Who do you need to forgive? How can you go about forgiving? What gesture can you make this week to forgive? (Examples: Make a phone call, write a letter, meet with them in person.) Remember, extending forgiveness is more about you and your freedom than the other person.
   _____
   _____
   _____
   _____
   _____

10. **Love like there is no tomorrow.**
    When you don't feel like being loving, how can you love anyway? What are some concrete actions you can take to show the people in your life that you love them? What is your love strength? What are your weak points in showing love? How will you work on it?
    _____
    _____
    _____
    _____
    _____

My Plan to Honor My Spiritual Self

Exercise time: 15 minutes

Spiritual practices come in all forms. Often, life gets so busy that we forget the spiritual practices that make us feel peaceful. Take about fifteen minutes to write freely about

Spiritual Health: Connecting Daily

what you intend to do to keep your spiritual life thriving. You can include time to attend your church, synagogue, temple or mosque. You can include time to read spiritual literature or sacred texts. Above, we explored prayer and meditation. Perhaps your spiritual practice includes meeting with a group of like-minded people who enjoy a similar spiritual practice. Or maybe it's to spend an entire day once weekly to commune with nature. Whatever it is, you can only heal completely when you take time for this aspect of yourself.

_____
_____
_____
_____
_____
_____
_____
_____
_____
_____
_____
_____
_____
_____
_____
_____

CHAPTER SEVEN

EMOTIONAL HEALTH & HEALING YOUR PAST

What you are feeling on a consistent basis truly dictates your health. If you go through your day feeling happy, vibrant and hopeful, the hormones and chemicals you create will keep you healthy. Inversely, when you are constantly feeling anxious, worried, or depressed, your body will create harmful chemicals and stress hormones.

While we don't always have control over what we feel, we do have control over what we do with those feelings. Do you allow the feelings to perpetuate or do you stop them dead in their tracks? Are you feeding off of negative energy or do you try to turn negative thoughts into positive ones?

In the following exercises, try to decipher what your emotional state is on a day-to-day basis and what you can do to change it if it's no longer serving you.

My Day Emotionally

Starting from the moment you wake up, mentally go through your day and notice what emotions come up as you envision each hour and activity you do or must do. Do you wake up happy, anxious or stressed? As you prepare for work, school or another morning activity, how do you feel? Close your eyes, and notice what comes up for each moment. Then, write down your answers next to each activity. For example, if you thought about your lunch and your feelings were "hungry" and "excited". Write it down. You will get an idea of whether your day is leaving you feeling more positive or more negative.

_____
_____
_____
_____
_____
_____
_____
_____
_____

Now that you've assessed your day emotionally, reread it. Wherever you notice a concentration of negative feelings put a check mark by it. Below, explain why you think you have negative feelings surrounding the subjects you checked. Explain also how you think you can change those things.

_____
_____
_____
_____
_____
_____
_____

My Stress Management Strategy Plan

How you manage stress will by and large determine your emotional health. If you process stress and stressful situations as highly emotionally charged, you will have a more difficult time taking control of your emotions. Below you will write ways in which you currently manage stress. Then you will add things you are willing to do to better manage your stress.

I manage stress now by… (Examples: taking a walk, drinking, smoking, going for a jog, venting, watching TV or playing video games etc.)
_____
_____
_____
_____
_____

These are ways I can manage stress, even though I may have not tried them yet… (Examples: deep breathing, meditation, listening to soothing music, going outdoors, screaming into a pillow, writing in a journal, dancing, throwing pebbles into a pond, painting, vacuuming, playing Legos with my kids etc.)
_____
_____
_____
_____
_____

You get to decide your emotional state each and every day. It's as easy as a choice. When you wake up in the morning, say aloud, "Today is going to be a fantastic day!" Then allow yourself to follow through.

Working through emotional states of your Ayurvedic mind body type

In *The Wheel of Healing with Ayurveda,* you learned in the chapter on Emotional Health that each dosha reacts and acts differently emotionally. It can be liberating to discover your propensity to act a certain way or feel a certain way based on your mind body type. This does not mean you are a prisoner to these emotions. On the contrary, it's a useful tool to detect when you are going out of balance. Remember, the idea in learning and mastering the principles of your Ayurvedic mind body type is to be able to bring yourself back into balance quickly. Reread the pages on *A Quick Guide to Rebalancing Your Emotional Body Through the Doshas*. Then write down how you normally find yourself reacting in relation to your most dominant mind body type.
_____
_____
_____

_____

_____

Learning From Your Past and Most Recent Past

Sometimes our past emotional states can hold us back though. Moving forward is a decision. Your body, mind, soul and spirit will be open to healing when you break the chains of past events that weigh you down. Try the following exercise whenever you feel the weight of your past.

"Sending flowers around it and letting it go."
Exercise time: 20-30 minutes

I once did some emotional work with a nurse practitioner, who lead me through the following exercise. You can use this exercise whenever you want to release emotions or let go of something from your past. You might want to have someone read it to you. Or you can record it and play it back so you can follow along without reading.

Find at least twenty minutes where you can sit quietly and comfortably in a private space.

Close your eyes and take a few deep breaths. First, think of your favorite place where you would go to relax. It could be a beach, a favorite vacation spot, or a special area in your garden or yard where you like to sit. When you are in this place you feel safe and secure. Imagine this place now. Notice how it feels to be there. Notice how your body feels calm. Your breathing is slow and relaxed. This is your safe spot. You can always return here whenever you start to feel uncomfortable.

Next, with your eyes closed and in the security of your safe space, bring to mind your natural thoughts and see what comes up. You are going to watch your thoughts like a movie reel. When thoughts arise, just watch them go by. Once a thought arises, it will float by and go away just the same. Notice if you engage a thought, it will stay for a longer time. But for right now, we are practicing observing. Just sit, watch and observe what comes up when you let your thoughts go.

With your eyes still closed, bring to mind an event of your past. The event could be happy, upsetting or neutral. Watch the event or the memory of the event just like you watched the other thoughts. Allow the memory to arise, pass by you like a movie reel and disappear from view.

Now, bring up a thought from the past that has been disturbing you for some time. It could involve a person, situation, circumstance or event. When you are thinking of this event, feel the emotions that arise with the thoughts. After a minute or so, imagine the most beautiful and fragrant flowers you've ever seen. Take those flowers and place them around your past event. Surround the people, place and your feelings with those flowers. And then, with beauty surrounding them, bid them goodbye and send them off. If you find yourself becoming too emotional, go back to your safe place for a moment. With your eyes still closed, feel the warmth and protection of your safe place.

Then, when you are feeling calmer and stronger, go to the next unpleasant memory that you would like to send away. Bring that memory to mind and once again, surround it with flowers after you have felt the fullness of the past impression. You can continue to do this as long as you have negative memories of your past that come up. Feel the emotions, send them flowers and let them go in the same way they arrived.

When your mind is clearer you can come back to your safe place once again. Feel the lightness in your body now that you have let go and said goodbye to those negative thoughts of the past. At one time, you needed those events. At one time, those events helped you grow. But now it's time to say good-bye and move forward knowing that those past impressions will not weigh you down anymore. You are free. You are light. You are empowered. Say to yourself, "I am free. I am light. I am empowered. I am free. I am light. I am empowered. I am free. I am light. I am empowered." When you are ready, you can slowly open your eyes.

You can use this exercise whenever you find yourself stuck thinking about a situation or person that is no longer serving you for the greater good.

The Only Limitations are the Ones Within Your Mind.

Strive to be limitless. The mind is powerful for good and for bad. One aspect of our past includes beliefs that we have adhered to. Many of those may limit the future. For example, I could not play sports well as a little girl. I was awkward and felt self conscious throwing a ball. In gym class, I was the last one to be chosen for a team. This made me feel unworthy in the sporting world. As an adult, if you were to ask me to play tennis, I might answer, "Oh, I'm not very good at it. I probably couldn't even hit the ball." This is a limitation I have put upon myself. Truth be told, there is no reason I couldn't play tennis. My arms are in fine working order and my heart is strong enough for the movement. Yet, because of my past experiences with sports, I have a notion that I wouldn't be any good. In order to be limitless, my response would need to change to, "Well, I haven't played tennis in a long time and I might be rusty. But I'd be willing to give it a try."

Do you have stories that limit you in some way today? How can you lift these to open yourself to infinite possibilities? What do you believe you can't do because of some past experience or words from someone in your past?

Lifting the Limits

Think of three things that you've thought about doing in the past but were stopped by a limiting mindset. What can you say to yourself to overcome the limitations you've put upon yourself? Write the excuse you have used in the past and then write your new affirmation for the present and future.

1.

2.

3.

CHAPTER EIGHT

RELATIONSHIP HEALTH

Connecting with others is one of the most rewarding aspects of our lives here on earth. As humans we are meant to be interdependent. This interdependence creates meaning that we cannot recreate alone. Think about the people who mean the most to you and how you can count on them to make your life more meaningful. In the following exercise, make a list of each person you would consider to be a close family member, a friend or significant other. Rate their level of importance to you. For example, if it is your child, you might rate him or her as number one or extremely important. Then, as you consider each of these people, write down what they bring to you, in qualities, to make your life richer.

Name of person	Relationship	Level of importance or significance	Ways he or she makes my life richer

In any of the relationships above, do you have friction or something you'd like to have resolved? If so, name the person, relationship and the issues below.

_____
_____
_____
_____
_____

As mentioned in *The Wheel of Healing with Ayurveda,* we first need to have a loving relationship with ourselves before we can expand to optimal relationships with others. It's difficult to ask our loved ones to be everything that we are not or that we need to be ourselves. In the following exercise, you are going to write yourself two love letters. The first love letter will be praise to everything you already are. Talk about your strengths in relationships. Explain in your letter what you're able to bring to another. In the second love letter, lovingly encourage yourself as to what you'd like to become in a relationship. For example, maybe jealously is an issue for you and you'd like to learn self-confidence to overcome it. Or maybe you're not as affectionate as you'd like to be. Another example might be the wish to be more mindful and less forgetful in a relationship.

My Love Letter to Myself

Dear _____,

_____
_____
_____
_____
_____
_____
_____
_____
_____
_____
_____
_____
_____
_____
_____
_____

My Love Letter to My Potential Self

Dear _____,

_____
_____
_____
_____
_____
_____
_____
_____
_____
_____
_____
_____

Now that you've written two love letters to yourself, reread the second one and then read through the *12 Traits to Healthy Relationships* in *The Wheel of Healing with Ayurveda*. Based on your second love letter, jot down the traits you would like to improve upon. For example, if you feel you could work on blaming less when something goes wrong, write it down. Or if you feel that the small stuff constantly bugs you and you find yourself nitpicking in relationships, write it down.

In the *12 Traits to Healthy Relationships*, I can improve upon the following:
_____
_____
_____
_____
_____

Next, look to your previous list about the things that are bothering you in some of your relationships. Match that list to the one above on what you'd like to improve in your own relationship health and notice if any of them are similar. Often, we see patterns in what we find wrong in our relationships and it comes back to what we'd like to improve in ourselves.

A Love Letter to My Most Significant Relationship

In this exercise, you are going to take one of the people you listed earlier in the chapter and write him or her a love letter. Just like you wrote for yourself in the first letter, write to this person all the traits you love about him or her. You can gush about great memories, the time you met or growing up together. Mention all the things you adore about this person. This should be a no-holds-barred letter. Let it flow and make the other person feel magnificent. Please stay positive in your letter. If you have more than one person you'd like to do this exercise for, you can repeat it on a separate sheet of paper. You may be tempted to write it on the computer, email or text. But in my experience letters written by hand, to loved ones, are the most cherished. Use the lines below as a template and then rewrite the letter and give it to your loved one.

Dear_____,
_____
_____
_____
_____
_____

Allowing Your Loved Ones to Shine Bright

Becoming the best version of you is the best way to ensure successful relationships. Strive to shift your focus away from changing others and work on becoming your best. In allowing yourself to become everything you want to be, you are allowing those you love the space to become better too. Many times we enter relationships hoping to change the other. This strategy almost never works. By being a guiding light through your own strength, you will allows others to shine brightly too. In closing this chapter, I'd like to share a story I once heard as an ancient tale, which shows that the wisdom of being your best self can help change others.

The Magic Paper

There was once a married couple that lived in a quiet village in a far away country. The woman, a fine wife, loved her husband but had a sharp tongue. The husband was a gruff man, loud and boisterous. It didn't take much to set off his anger. He was proud and harsh. His words were often cutting and rude. His wife did not take to his words gently. She often spoke back to him in a loud tone, and told him he should treat her more kindly. She contradicted what he said on a regular basis. This made the husband angrier and his gruffness grew worse with her disrespect. Needless to say, the married couple was in a bit of trouble.

The wife, desperate, went to visit the town sage, an older woman down the road. She told the old lady of her troubles. As she spoke, the old woman simply nodded and began to fold up a piece of paper. Weary and in tears, the wife cried out, "Can you help me? I want to save my marriage but I cannot live any longer with this loud and boisterous man." The old woman folded the last bit of paper, which was now a tiny rectangle no bigger than a tooth. She held the paper out to the weary wife and said, "My dear, take this magic paper. Place it in between your back teeth. Every time your husband shows his anger, bite on it, hard. Then smile and nod. The more he shouts, the harder you will bite." Shocked, the wife looked up and said, "But how will this help my marriage? I asked you to give me advice." The old woman just nodded her head and gestured to the paper in her hand and said, "Take it. Now go."

Incredulous, the wife took the paper and stormed out of the old lady's home. Soon after, the husband returned demanding his supper and complaining about his day as usual. The wife began to shout out, "Your day? Would you believe..."But then she stopped. Quickly looking down at the paper, she stuffed it between her back teeth and bit hard. The husband continued to shout and she continued to bite the paper. Within minutes the husband stopped shouting and walked away.

The next day, the same thing occurred. The husband came home in a foul mood and his stream of demands filled the air. The wife bit the paper, smiled and nodded. Within a couple of minutes, the husband was silent. He left her presence with a sigh and his anger seemed to melt away.

By the fifth day, the husband entered the home a little differently. He had picked some wildflowers on the way and instead of stomping in the house, the way he normally did, he came in a little more quietly. Upon seeing his wife, he held out the wildflowers and immediately left to wash up for dinner without a word.

On the seventh day of the magic paper, the husband ran in through the door and went directly to his wife. He picked her up, spun her around and kissed her tenderly on the lips. And these were the words he spoke to her, "My wife, I had forgotten how beautiful you are. Your hair glistens in the sunlight and your smile is brighter than any I have ever seen. I am so proud that you are my wife."

The next morning, the wife returned to see the old lady. And she said to her, "It is a miracle. This magic paper works. My husband has become a loving man once again. Please dear lady, tell me of this magic so that I may have it forever."

The old lady looked into the woman's eyes, this woman who was so sad just one week ago and said to her, "My dear, don't you understand? The paper did nothing but help you keep your mouth shut. It is you who changed your husband by being the loving wife you once were. Your husband reacts to the way you are inside. Your silence allowed you to be more loving and kind. Your silence helped you to not judge and criticize. Your silence allowed him to see your beauty. The way you were, transformed him into the man you wanted him to be."

CHAPTER NINE

OCCUPATIONAL, FINANCIAL *and* ENVIRONMENTAL HEALTH

In The Wheel of Healing with Ayurveda, I divided these three aspects of health into separate chapters. As they are interrelated, we will explore these together in this workbook. To create the life of your dreams, visualization is a helpful tool. For most of us, much of our time is consumed with career and finances. The environments that surround us are in direct correlation with our job and our financial status. Many of us live in a certain geographical location because our job is there. And the neighborhood, you choose to live in, is either influenced by job location, finances or both.

Remember, you don't need to limit your concept of environment to your immediate geographical surroundings. You environment includes your workplace or workspace, your car, the space inside your home and also the people you live with or who surround you on a constant basis.

It's easy to overlook factors such as work, money and environment when it comes to your health. But they are strong influencing factors in your wellbeing.

While we may strive to be satisfied in all three of these areas equally, the truth is that one or two of these may take priority. For example, let's suppose you have a great job that you love and that pays well, but is in a cold climate and you hate the cold. Or perhaps you are in your dream location but the jobs there are mediocre at best.

Take a moment now and prioritize in order of preference between job, money and location or environment.

1. _____
2. _____
3. _____

Once you've made the decision between the three as to the most important, you can make more effort to create changes in your top priority first. This certainly does not mean that you can't have it all. It does, however, give you a starting point.

Using Visualization and Vision Boards to Create Your Life

If you can imagine it, you can achieve it. If you can dream it, you can become it.
-William A. Ward.

That quote, printed on a poster, which hung on my bedroom closet, was one that I saw every day of my childhood. And I believe that quote helped me become the person I am today.

Generally, what's in front of us, we move toward. We bring into our environment that which we see daily and that which is familiar to us. Creating a vision board gives you a real picture of what you want to create in your life.

You don't need to be artistic to create a vision board. As humans we tend to naturally think visually. If I ask you to close your eyes and envision a chocolate cake, could you do it? My bet is yes.

If you are to move toward the job you want, the financial status you desire and the environment you long for, you need to start retraining your brain to think in terms of those things rather than what you are experiencing now.

Start with your number one on the list above. Imagine what would make it great for you. For example, if you wrote money as your number one, think about what financial status you'd like to attain. What would be your annual income, the amount in your savings and investments? What would your lifestyle look like? What would you do in your spare time? How would you spend your money? How would it make you feel? What's the number you'd like to see in your bank daily? In pictures, what does money look like or the status of having money look like?

Or if environment is your number one, in what location would you choose to live? What does it look like? What is the climate? What kind of home would you live in? What does that look like? How would that make you feel? Who would live with you or close to you? What environment would surround your home? What might the landscape be? How would you use this ultimate environment in leisure time? What colors would describe it best?

Now, if job or occupation is your number one, what is your ideal job? What is the salary? What are your hours? What kind of people do you work with? What does your workspace look like? What are your duties and responsibilities? How does this job make you feel? How much vacation time do you receive per year? Who would you help and serve? What does the building look like, if any?

A Picture is Worth a Thousand Words

Once you've visualized your ideal job, financial status or environment, it's time to create your vision board.

Using a poster board, a corkboard or foam board, or you can create a digital vision board. I like the idea of physical vision boards because they require a mind body connection because of the physical work involved. However, for practicality, you may want to create one on your computer or smartphone. One website that is community based is called DreamItAlive. And you can also create a secret board on Pinterest. Writer, Jack Canfield has a smartphone app called *Success Vision Board,* which is free.

Gather pictures, images and quotes which represent your dreams. This portion of the exercise may take some time as you begin to think about your goals in pictures.

Adding Your Intentions and Desires

Once your images are in place, you can insert your intentions in your own words below each picture. In *The Wheel of Healing with Ayurveda* we learned how to create a list of intentions and desires. Keep the wording in your intentions positive. Keep your intentions in the present tense as if they are already in your life. And finally, phrase your intentions with gratitude to the universe for allowing your dreams to become reality.

Examples of intention and desires:
I am so happy and grateful to have achieved perfect health.
It is my intention to find the perfect mate for me.
I am happy and grateful to live within walking distance of the Pacific Ocean.
I am grateful to experience wealth and prosperity every day.
It is my intention to get hired in my dream job within three months from today.

Now that you have an idea of how to create your intentions and desires, write at least ten that will go along with your vision board.

My Intentions and Desires

_____
_____
_____
_____
_____
_____
_____
_____
_____
_____

CHAPTER TEN

AYURVEDA Q & A

Below you will find the answers to commonly asked questions about Ayurveda and living in balance with *The Wheel of Healing*.

Q: I have done the Mind Body Type test but I still don't know my dominant dosha or my prakruti. How do I find out?
A: Self-awareness is not an easy thing. Sometimes we are out of touch with who we really are. Other times we have pushed away our true nature for so long that we begin to believe we are someone who we are not. A good way to find out your prakruti is to do the dosha test with someone who knows you very well. You answer the prompt and your loved one will answer the prompt about you. Average out the scores between you and talk about the answers if you really don't agree about certain ones. But let me suffice it to say this; if you are angry and upset that the dosha test did not meet your expectations, you are a Pitta type. If you are anxious that you are not choosing the right answers and are having a hard time choosing, you are a Vata type. And if you are slow at comprehending the prompts and are beginning to not really care what the answers are, you are a likely to be a Kapha type.

Q: What if I scored the same for two doshas?
A: Even if two doshas are close, there is always a dominant dosha. Here is my rule of thumb: when you go out of balance throughout your life, you have a tendency to go out of balance with your dominant dosha first. Write down the symptoms you typically have when you go out of balance and see what dosha they fall under. Let me give you an example. A Vata type will tend to get nervous, stressed, fidgety, and get constipation. These are all symptoms of Vata. So it's probable that the Vata dosha is dominant.

Q: What if I am a Kapha type but my spouse is a Vata type? How do I cook the same meal for both of us?
A: The goal in Ayurvedic cooking is to make sure you integrate all six tastes at every meal. There should be a variety of foods within the same meal. Remember, according to your mind body type, you will have different proportions of the six tastes on your plate. If it's a question of flavoring or spices that may aggravate a Pitta type, for example, opt to keep the spices out of the dish and each person can add spices according to taste. A Kapha type will need more bitter, pungent and astringent tastes while a Vata type will need more sweet, sour and salty tastes. This can be easily rectified in a family by making a salad with more bitter, pungent and astringent and a main dish with all six tastes focusing a little more on the sweet, sour and salty tastes. In this meal, the Kapha type will eat more of the salad and less of the main dish and the Vata type will eat less of the salad and more of the main dish.

Q: What if my work schedule changes often? How do I stick with my Ayurvedic daily routine?
A: Try to stick with your Ayurvedic daily routine the best you can during your changing work times. For example, if you work late, aim to wake up early instead of sleeping in. It's easy to get caught up in a sleep cycle that goes against the circadian rhythm. If you work nights, do your daily routine at the time you wake up as if it's early morning.

Q: What about trying other diets while I'm living an Ayurvedic Lifestyle?
A: Learning how to eat a balanced and holistic diet can be challenging enough. Then add learning a diet to balance your dosha. It can get confusing if you add another diet to the mix. In my experience, many of the fad diets out there are restrictive. They either exclude an entire major food group or limit it to an extreme. The problem with extreme diets is that they are difficult to maintain and often can leave you out of balance in one or more of the doshas. By following an Ayurvedic Lifestyle Eating Plan, you will be eating healthier, in accordance with nature and balancing your mind body type. Since Ayurveda has been around for over 5,000 years, it has credibility too.

Q: Could it be that meditation is not for me? I've tried meditation several times and I have a hard time sitting still.
A: This may come as a surprise to you but most people cannot sit still unless they are occupied, entertained or asleep. So you are not alone! Practicing meditation like learning to drive, play golf or perfect the piano takes skill and a lot of practice. You are not expected to master it in a few sessions. When you meditate, you are training your brain to slow down. You are training your body to sit still in silence. This does not happen overnight. First, you must learn with a skilled teacher. Second, give yourself 90-days of consistent practice to develop meditation as a habit and build your meditation muscle, so to speak. Finally, if sitting still really is the challenge, build up your tolerance for sitting in silence. Start meditating for five minutes and then add a minute a day or every few days until you have reached thirty minutes. In a short time, you will find it easy and rewarding.

Q: When I meditate, my mind races with too many thoughts and some of them are disturbing. How can I quiet my mind and feel comfortable enough with all of these thoughts?
A: Just know that the nature of the mind is to think thoughts. It's nothing personal, that's just its job. With a regular meditation practice, especially a mantra-based meditation practice, you will notice your thoughts quiet down. Sometimes emotions will come up as a beginning meditator. Know that this is normal. Think about it, throughout your life, you've focused on the outer world. It's not often that we take time to get silent and focus on the world within. So when you start, the mind says, "Hey, it's my time now to bring up these things she hasn't yet resolved." As a result, you may feel inundated with thoughts and emotions. If this becomes troublesome, go back to the guided meditation exercise in chapter seven of this *Companion Workbook* and go through it or have someone read it to you. You can also journal your thoughts. In the end, this is a good thing. You are detoxifying your emotional body and becoming healthier instead of being afraid. It's time to celebrate!

Q: What if I want to get off my prescription pills? How long will it take before I can do that?
A: It can be frustrating when you must take prescription pills. And often many of these prescriptions don't work optimally or give you side effects. When you add aspects of an Ayurvedic lifestyle, many symptoms and illnesses do subside and much of the time, disappear. This is the Ayurvedic principle of balance versus imbalance. Working with your healthcare practitioner, you can both determine what's best for your health and your situation. As an Ayurvedic practitioner, I have seen clients lower their blood pressure in

three weeks of meditation, level off their blood sugar with a daily yoga practice and lose weight as a result of eating an Ayurvedic diet.

That being said, there are certain prescription medications, such as psychotropic drugs (for anxiety, depression, or other mental illnesses), which take time to wean off of. Explain to your physician what you are doing to improve your health and see what his or her plan is for either lowering your medication doses or cutting them out altogether. If you find that your healthcare provider is not taking the time to consider your needs or is not open to integrative healthcare practices, you may need to switch doctors until you find one with a more open mind.

Q: Will Ayurveda help cure my alcohol and/or drug addiction(s)?
A: Many drugs, once they've crossed the blood-brain barrier over a period of time will create a chemical dependency. Alcohol is one of these drugs as are several street drugs and some prescription medications. Stopping a drug on which you are chemically dependent can be harmful to your health by causing seizures, strokes or cardiac arrest. If you believe you might be addicted to any of the above, it's best to contact an addiction specialist first and go through a proper detox program with medical supervision. What you will learn in a program is that chemical addictions to alcohol and drugs cannot be cured; they can only be arrested. Once you are in an addiction treatment program after detox, living an Ayurvedic lifestyle can be a wonderful way to help keep you sober and clean for years to come. The connection between mind, body, soul and spirit is what you will need to have the strength to get and stay sober.

Q: The concepts in Ayurveda seem rather simple and trivial. Does it really work?
A: Going back to the basics is where most of us need to be. Our lives and health have become too complicated. Read over the principles of health, exercise, meditation or quiet reflection, emotional health, and assess these few things. Are you doing most of them on a daily basis? If the answer is "no", try these first with complete dedication and see if your health improves. There are more complex aspects of Ayurvedic medicine but in my practice I have found that most people are not paying attention to the simple things that will improve their health exponentially.

Q: Can Ayurveda help get rid of certain illnesses?
A: Yes, with the help of an experienced practitioner. As mentioned in *The Wheel of Healing with Ayurveda*, there are six stages of disease according to Ayurveda. Full-blown illness is the sixth stage out of six. And so the imbalances that occurred to reach that stage had been occurring for a while. Some diseases are the cause of one specific dosha being out of balance but many diseases, such as cancer, are multi-doshic. While much of

Ayurveda is preventative, there is a curative aspect of Ayurveda that is especially helpful when you are working with an Ayurvedic practitioner. And most often, you will also be working in conjunction with your allopathic healthcare provider.

Q: Ayurveda is considered to be timeless and eternal, why is that?
A: While trends, lifestyles and knowledge may change, the building blocks of the human body and the surrounding elements have not changed. Since Ayurveda works with the building blocks of nature, one can apply its principles in any time period. Ayurveda was a science before formal science was discovered. It is the only medical science, which has lasted for over 5,000 years and has proven to be effective in preventive and curative health.

CHAPTER ELEVEN

SIMPLE MEAL PLANS *for* VATA, PITTA, & KAPHA

You can get started quickly on your dosha-specific diet with a few menu suggestions for each dosha below. Each menu choice has all six tastes represented in each meal with the appropriate proportions of each taste for Vata, Pitta and Kapha. In all of these choices, you will still follow *The 12 Guidelines to an Ayurvedic Lifestyle Eating Plan* and *The 10 Guidelines to Eating Awareness* as explained in *The Wheel of Healing with Ayurveda.*

Vata Pacifying Breakfast Choices

Menu Choice 1: Cream of wheat or cream of rice made with 2% milk. Stir in a pinch of salt, cinnamon, cardamom, and/or nutmeg. To sweeten, add a tablespoon of maple syrup and for a smooth flavor, add a teaspoon of ghee or butter if desired. Add five soaked raw almonds (soaked overnight) with or without the skins. To top the hot cereal, you can add fresh blueberries or strawberries. Drink a hot tea (either black or green) with lemon and honey or instead add a dash of cardamom to the tea. (Coffee is generally not recommended for a Vata type while balancing, although decaffeinated coffee may be O.K.)

Menu Choice 2: Two organic eggs scrambled made with butter or olive oil with ½ ounce of cheese, flavored with salt and pepper topped with fresh sliced tomato and cilantro. Add a whole grain English muffin with butter or ghee and a veggie sausage. Complete the meal with a glass of fresh squeezed orange juice.

Vata Pacifying Lunch Choices

Menu Choice 1: A hearty cream-based soup such as broccoli and cheddar or potato soup. Add a slice of whole grain bread with organic butter or olive oil. Have a hot apple cobbler for dessert. Drink warm or hot water with lemon.

Menu Choice 2: Asian vegetable stir-fry (carrots, sugar snap peas, broccoli, zucchini, bell peppers, onions, ginger, garlic) with chicken breast or tofu served with steamed brown rice. Drink warm or hot water with lemon.

Vata Pacifying Dinner Choices

Menu Choice 1: Whole-wheat pasta, drizzled with extra virgin olive oil, topped with sautéed spinach, zucchini, bell peppers, onions and garlic. Add grated parmesan or pecorino cheese. Add a slice whole grain garlic bread with organic butter or olive oil. Drink a Vata herbal tea or hot water with lemon.

Menu Choice 2: Lightly sautéed trout in olive oil or butter, topped with toasted almonds and served with herb butter (made with dill, parsley and cilantro) mashed potatoes and lightly steamed then sautéed green beans. Add a bread pudding for desert. Drink a Vata herbal tea or hot water with lemon.

Vata Pacifying Snacks

With the Vata snacks, you can make combinations to get all six tastes.

2% Greek yogurt with honey or jam
Cooked apple with cinnamon, nutmeg and brown sugar
A ripe pear, mango, apricot, peach or banana
An organic cheese stick
A slice of fresh whole grain bread with peanut or a nut butter
Sliced avocado with a teaspoon of olive oil and a dash of salt

Pitta Pacifying Breakfast Choices

Menu Choice 1: Green smoothie made with 2 cups of baby kale or spinach, 2 cups of coconut water or coconut milk, 3 cups of a combination of banana, mango, berries, oranges, apples, pineapples or grapes. You can also add cinnamon, cardamom, flax seeds or almond butter to your smoothie. Make sure you blend the leafy greens with the coconut water before you add the fruit to get a smooth taste. You can freeze a banana ahead of time to get a colder smoothie without using ice.

Menu Choice 2: Homemade fruit and nut granola made with dried cherries, cranberries, pumpkin seeds, sunflower seeds, and almonds with skim organic milk and topped with fresh berries. Add a small side of greek yogurt with honey. Drink a cup of Pitta pacifying tea or a green mint tea.

Pitta Pacifying Lunch Choices

Menu Choice 1: (for two people) Mix two Belgian endives sliced into thin slices with ½ cup of toasted organic walnuts (chopped), one golden apple (peeled and cut into cubes), add ¼ cup of crumbled blue cheese. Top with a homemade vinaigrette dressing of one tablespoon of Champagne vinegar, mix with one teaspoon of Dijon mustard, add salt and pepper to taste. Then mix in two tablespoons of extra virgin olive oil. Add a slice of whole grain bread with butter or olive oil. Drink room temperature water.

Menu Choice 2: Homemade taboulé style salad made with one cup of organic bulgur wheat soaked in one cup of boiling water and left to cool. Chop three fresh Roma tomatoes, one cucumber (peeled and seeded), one sweet onion, one bunch of curly parsley, and a handful of fresh mint leaves. If you enjoy the sweet taste, you can also add ¼ cup of golden raisins. Mix ingredients and top with a dressing of the juice from one to two lemons, ¼ cup of extra virgin olive oil, one crushed and finely chopped garlic clove and salt and pepper to taste. Drink room temperature water.

Pitta Pacifying Dinner Choices

Menu Choice 1: Grilled tuna steak with herbs de Provence and served with a cilantro pesto sauce, roasted rosemary red skin potatoes and grilled asparagus. Served with a chilled cucumber soup on the side.

Menu Choice 2: Grilled vegetable fajitas made with grilled Portobello mushrooms, green peppers, onions, and zucchini. Add whole-wheat flour tortillas, fresh guacamole, mild pico de gallo (or a mango salsa), a small dollop of sour cream, and a mild cheese such as Monterey jack or a mild cheddar. Grill corn on the cob on the side.

Pitta Pacifying Snacks

With the Pitta snacks, you can make combinations to get all six tastes. Although according to Ayurveda, melons should be eaten alone.

Fresh watermelon or cantaloupe
Fresh mangoes, ripe bananas, pears or apples
A fresh berry salad mixed with chopped fresh mint leaves and drizzled with honey or maple syrup
Fresh carrots, celery, cucumbers, bell peppers, mushrooms dipped in hummus
Edamame
Mango or rose lassi with cardamom

Kapha Pacifying Breakfast Choices

Menu Choice 1: 3/4 cup dry cereal without added sugar: Ezekiel 4:9 brand, cereal, Uncle Sam cereal, or Shredded wheat cereal. Add one cup of room temperature unsweetened almond milk, one cup of mixed berries: raspberries, blackberries, blueberries, strawberries, and one cup black coffee or herbal tea with a pinch of ground cloves to add pungency.

Menu Choice 2: One egg plus one egg white omelet made with olive oil cooking spray and some of the following veggies: peppers, spinach, onions, cilantro, parsley, tomatoes, mushrooms, chili peppers, one veggie sausage & one Ezekiel brand English muffin or one small whole-wheat tortilla, a cup black coffee or herbal tea with a pinch of ground cloves.

Menu Choice 3: One cup hot oatmeal or hot, whole grain cereal made with, unsweetened almond milk, pinch of salt and cinnamon, nutmeg or cloves, topped with a choice of 1/2 cup blueberries, raspberries, or blackberries (If you need to sweeten, add 1 tsp of honey or maple syrup). One cup black coffee or herbal tea.

Kapha Pacifying Lunches

Menu Choice 1: Veggie wrap made with an Ezekiel 4:9 brand sprouted grain tortilla with any or all of the following: hummus, leafy greens, spinach, cilantro, carrots, peppers, mushrooms, cucumbers, sprouts. On the side: raw veggies: carrots, celery, radishes, broccoli, cauliflower dipped in 2 TB of Genji All-Natural Ginger Miso dressing. Drink warm water, ginger or green tea.

Menu Choice 2: Veggie Burger on a whole wheat bun, Dijon mustard, sprouts, lettuce, tomato, 1/4 avocado, 1 tsp mayonnaise (if desired). Raw veggies with Ginger Miso Dressing. Drink green or herbal tea.

Menu Choice 3: Greek style salad made with cucumbers, grape tomatoes, bell peppers, 6 Kalamata olives, 2 TB of feta cheese, 1/4 cup chick peas (garbanzo beans), 1 TB of each: fresh dill, cilantro, parsley. Top with a dressing of 2 TB fresh lemon juice, 2 tsp olive oil, 1 garlic clove, crushed salt, pepper to taste. Ten multigrain-style pita chips with ¼ cup of hummus. Drink green or herbal tea.

Kapha Pacifying Dinners

Menu Choice 1: Minestrone style soup made with red kidney beans, green beans, one fennel bulb, one zucchini, three cloves of garlic, one onion, freshly chopped parsley, freshly chopped basil, red pepper flakes, oregano, Italian herbs, tomato paste, and vegetable broth. Use a minimal amount of olive oil when cooking and limit the salt but add pepper to taste.

Menu Choice 2: Grilled salmon salad made with blackened grilled fresh salmon, arugula, fresh chopped fennel, orange slices, ¼ avocado, and cilantro. You don't even need a dressing for this salad since the juice from the orange slices with give it some moisture. But if you prefer, you can add freshly squeezed lime juice, a teaspoon of olive oil, salt and pepper to taste.

GLOSSARY *of* SANSKRIT TERMS

abhyanga: Daily oil massage.

akasha: Space or ether.

ama: A toxic residue caused by undigested food, experiences, and emotions. The term translates as "toxins in the body and mind."

artha: Material wealth, gain, or prosperity. One of the four goals in life that are known, in Vedic morality, as the purusharthas.

asana: A yoga pose.

Ayurveda: The science of life; the name is derived from the Sanskrit words ayus, meaning "life," and veda, meaning "science or knowledge."

chakras: The energy centers in the body, related to the nerve plexus centers. There are seven main chakras, which together align the spine.

Charaka Samhita: An early text on Ayurveda. The Charaka Samhita and the Sushruta Samhita are the two foundational texts of this field; both date to the early centuries of the common era.

dharma: An individual's purpose in life.

dosha: The three main psychophysiological principles of the body (Vata, Pitta, Kapha), which determine a person's individual mind-body constitution.

ghee: Clarified butter.

gunas: one of the three qualities of nature or *prakruti*, which are *sattva*, *rajas* and *tamas*.

Kapha: One of the three doshas, it combines the elements water and earth. It is responsible for bodily structure.

karma: Action or deed. It is also the principle of causality, in which a person's intent in taking an action in the present equals a particular result in the future.

jala: Water.

mahabhutas: The great elements: space, air, fire, water, and earth.

mantra: Derived from two Sanskrit words: man, meaning "mind," and tra, meaning "instrument." This instrument of the mind is a sound or series of sounds used to connect body, mind, and spirit.

nasya: Method of administering oil or herbalized oil to the nostrils. It is one of the five parts of panchakarma.

ojas: Healing chemicals in the body that are by-products of properly digested food, emotions, and experiences.

Pitta: The biological humor in Ayurveda composed of the elements fire and water.

prakruti: The biological constitution of an individual. It is determined at conception and is composed of certain proportions of the three doshas: Vata, Pitta, and Kapha.

prana: Vital life energy, or life force.

pranayama: Yogic breathing techniques; also, the fourth branch of yoga.

prithivi: The earth element.

rajas: passion (one of the three gunas)

rishis: Ancient sages, or seers, from India.

sattva: goodness or purity (one of the three gunas)

Surya Namaskar: Sun Salutations, a series of yoga poses that coordinate with the breath.

tamas (tamasic): dullness or inertia (one of the three gunas)

tejas: Fire.

Vata: Composed of space and air, this is one of the three doshas, or Ayurvedic mind-body types.

vayu: Wind or air.

vikruti: The current state of an individual, in contrast to a person's natural state, or prakruti. This state may indicate imbalances in an individual's mind-body constitution.

yoga: Derived from the Sanskrit word yuj, which means "to yoke" or "to join together." In yoga, we join together our mind, body, soul, and spirit.

If you enjoyed *The Wheel of Healing with Ayurveda: An Easy Guide to a Healthy Lifestyle* and *The Wheel of Healing with Ayurveda Companion Workbook,* check out:
Secrets of The Wheel of Healing 8-CD Audio Course with Workbook

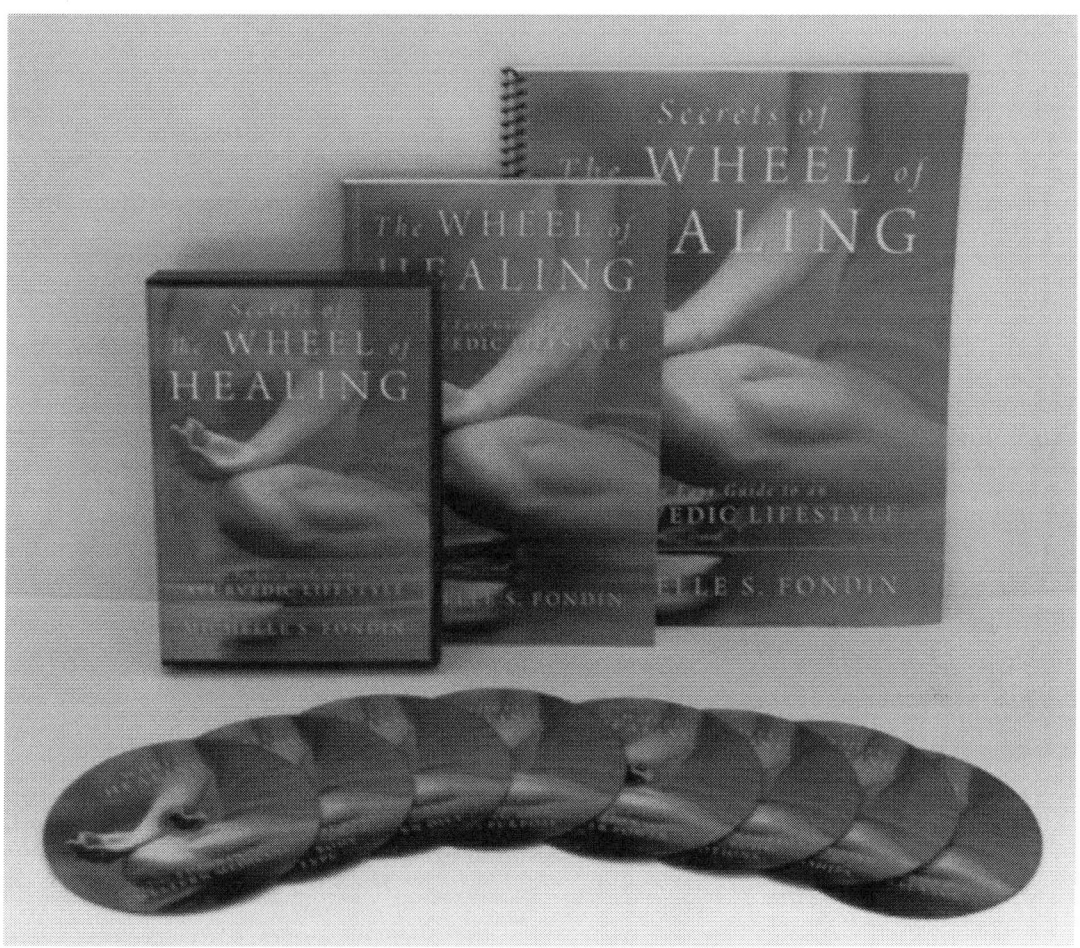

For this and other products go to:
www.thewheelofhealing.com
Contact the author:
contact@michellefondin.com
To book Michelle Fondin for an event, write to:
events@michellefondin.com

Made in United States
Troutdale, OR
12/22/2023